The BE CLEAR Method to Living with Bronchiectasis

A self-care guide to improving lung health and general well-being

Linda Cooper Esposito, MPH

To Tony

CONTENTS

" *Our bodies are our gardens to which our wills are gardeners.*

WILLIAM SHAKESPEARE

" *Learning to treat ourselves lovingly may at first feel like a dangerous experiment.*

SHARON SALZBERG

WHY I WROTE THIS GUIDE

There are many books about asthma and COPD and a number of them are written from a personal perspective. This is not the case for the chronic lung disease that I have, bronchiectasis. I decided to fill the void with this book, *The BE CLEAR Method to Living with Bronchiectasis*, hoping others will relate, gain a deeper understanding of the disease and be uplifted.

In the past, bronchiectasis was often misdiagnosed and misunderstood. That is changing, and BE (a short way of saying bronchiectasis) is now considered the third most common reason for chronic airway disease. Some physicians and researchers speculate that due to the COVID-19 pandemic, we will see a steady increase in bronchiectasis cases worldwide.

Bronchiectasis, the irreversible scarring of the airway passages, is a lifelong condition. Although I am an upbeat, optimistic person, I am also a realist—I trust evidence-based research. Presenting the facts about bronchiectasis is one of the main goals of this guide. You might hear anecdotal stories about complete healing, but research in adults with BE continues to show that the condition is permanent.

My second goal is to lay out a way for readers to actively participate in maintaining optimal health. When I use the term "optimal health," I am speaking on an individual level as people with bronchiectasis make up a heterogeneous group. Some of us have scarring from previous infections, others from underlying genetic conditions. Within such a varied group, optimal health will look different for each person.

Even with our differences, we all share a need to break the cycle of mucus production, inflammation, infection, and bronchiectasis disease progression. We can disrupt this cycle by practicing daily self-care to create a healing environment in our bodies. This guide shares with you my approach to self-care and gives you suggestions for yours. It is a template for you to create a self-care healing plan and a jumping-off point for discussions with your medical team.

Self-care alone might not be enough for you to control your infection; antibiotics and other pharmacological interventions might be necessary. The steps outlined here can be taken in conjunction with medications or in their absence.

Most importantly, we are a community seeking optimal health for all. Just as a flower blooms without comparing itself to other flowers, so should we. Let's grow as a community in our knowledge and our commitment to doing our part in managing our chronic condition.

MY STORY AND THE BE CLEAR METHOD

In the fall of 2017, I received an upsetting phone call. It went something like this:

"Your CT scan shows bronchiectasis."

"Bron-key-eck-ta-sis," I repeated haltingly. "What is it?"

"Scarring of the lung airways," my doctor said, adding, "probably caused by a bacterial infection. Let's get you a consultation with a pulmonologist."

"Sure," I said, trying to take it all in calmly. "Sounds like a plan."

I hung up the phone in disbelief. I have a Master's in Public Health from Yale, had worked in medical facilities for years and was familiar with many respiratory conditions, but not bronchiectasis. I wondered if this mysterious disease could be the reason for my chronic cough.

For almost a year, I'd believed that my cough was due to silent acid reflux. My doctor had prescribed medication to reduce the acid in my stomach that was supposedly making me cough. Always the good student, I had amassed a stack of books on acid reflux by my bedside— The Acid Watcher Diet, Dr. Koufman's Acid Reflux Diet and The

Chronic Cough. I had given up coffee, spicy foods, pickles and wine. None of that seemed to have made a difference. I was beginning to understand why.

The pulmonologist explained that bronchiectasis was a rare disease and from my CT scan, I probably also had a rare infection called Mycobacterium Avium Complex (MAC). This was later confirmed by sputum analysis. Before leaving the doctor's office, a nurse showed me how to use an Aerobika®, a hand-held device that clears mucus out of airways. I'd told her mine was a dry cough and that I did not have any mucus. Even so, she told me to try my best to clear out what might be there anyway. After a brief time practicing with the Aerobika, the receptionist scheduled me for a follow-up appointment. In a daze, I walked to the crosstown bus stop while phoning my husband.

I stood swaying with the bus as it took the curve westward through Central Park. The pulmonologist had assured me that I was not contagious, but still, I did my best not to cough on anyone near me. With my fellow New Yorkers pressing against me, I felt despondent and alone with my thoughts.

Gazing out the window, I saw the familiar cracks in the park's retaining wall with the tree roots breaking through to find light on that crisp October afternoon. I too was trying to find light, to find clarity. Using a mindfulness practice I'd learned in college, I focused on the surface of the winding park wall and as anxiety crept into my mind, I tried to gently push it aside.

I hopped off the bus near ABC Studios to walk the last half mile home. New York City makes it easy to stay fit. Getting around often means walking, walking… and more walking. Not to mention the steep flights of subway steps that are better than any stair-climbing machine at the gym.

I moved to New York City in 1997 from a Connecticut suburb during a difficult period in my first marriage. I had left my position as a health administrator and was suffering from anxiety and back pain. I did what came naturally and immediately joined a neighborhood gym. I took strength training and yoga classes but, most of all, I loved what was at the time a new exercise concept–Pilates. On the studio wall above the exercise equipment was a framed quote from the creator of the method, Joseph Pilates, "Change happens through movement and movement heals." As I stretched and worked my muscles, I felt as if Mr. Pilates were speaking directly to me. Over time, I enrolled in a personal trainer certification program. I loved studying the body. I started to incorporate what I was learning into my own workouts and my ever-present anxiety and back pain noticeably improved.

As a fitness and health educator, I found myself seeking out clients with chronic conditions. I've always loved a challenge, so coaching those who were terrified of exercise was right up my alley. My clients had conditions that ran the gamut—breast cancer, osteoporosis, back pain, depression—and had been told by their doctors that the best thing they could do for themselves was to exercise. Many were in their 60s and 70s and had never seen the inside of a gym. It was my job to get them stronger and to the point where "exercise" was no longer a scary word.

How ironic to find myself in a similar situation after my own diagnosis! I exercised regularly, but if I were being completely honest, I had slacked off. I was then approaching my retirement years and had—knowingly or unknowingly—put myself on what could best be described as a maintenance plan: a little yoga, a little Pilates, occasional strength training and perhaps a brisk walk along the Hudson River or in Central Park now and again. Before being diagnosed with bronchiectasis, I'd ignored my laid-back attitude and had even gone as far as justifying it. After all, I had exercised most of my life and now, remarried and living in New York City, I had other priorities that seemed more compelling than yet another yoga class or mindless miles on the treadmill. It struck me that the party was over. It was time for me to become my own client!

Before going home, I made a quick stop at the neighborhood grocery store. I wanted to make a pot of soup, something I did when feeling run down. I was not a fancy cook, but I was a healthy one. Loaded down with grocery bags, I went home to start my new life living with bronchiectasis.

In the kitchen, I fought back tears as I chopped vegetables. They fell as much from anger and disbelief about my diagnosis as from the onions. Amongst family and friends, I had a reputation for being a bit of a germaphobe. For example, if one of my daughters were having a party, as soon as the guests filled their plates, I would try to refrigerate what was left of the food. With my public health background, I knew that food left on a buffet table for hours was an open invitation for bacteria growth and food poisoning. "Mom, people may want seconds" or "We are still expecting a few stragglers" were often my daughters' ways of politely telling me to *leave the food alone!*

Yet again, the irony was glaring. The bacteria that had scarred my lungs had not come from left-out shrimp cocktail or potato salad. Instead, according to my pulmonologist, it most likely had come from the garden I'd maintained during the years after we moved out of Manhattan and relocated to Woodstock, New York.

While living upstate, I'd embraced gardening with exuberance and got through the frigid winter months by dreaming about new plantings. As soon as the ground thawed, I would get to work cleaning the flower beds and spreading wheelbarrows full of rich, nutritious mulch. I was in heaven. Now, with my bronchiectasis diagnosis and my doctor thinking that the MAC bacteria in the mulch and soil had contributed to my disease, I felt betrayed by my passion. How could gardening have made me so sick when I loved it so much?

The evening following my visit to the pulmonologist, my husband saw me moping around the apartment. "What's wrong?" he asked. "What's *not* wrong, you mean," I shot back, sharing with him how frightened and angry I was about my diagnosis. "Look at it this way," he said. "You've been taking such good care of yourself for so long. That has to make a difference. It's like money in the bank."

I thought about what he'd said. I had always been so healthy and now, having a condition that my doctor said would be with me for the rest of my life was a blow to the gut. I was angry, and when I'm angry, I take action. Trying to clear my lungs with the little gizmo the nurse had given me, the Aerobika, was a starting point. My online research had reinforced the importance of ridding my lungs of harmful mucus. Luckily, I connected with a support group leader through National Jewish Health, a leading respiratory hospital in Denver, Colorado. Speaking with the upbeat advocate, I knew I had hit the jackpot. She had been managing her bronchiectasis for over twenty years and attributed her success to airway clearance, exercise and a positive attitude. Well, I did not have an "I've got this" attitude yet, but I could try to kick butt with airway clearance and exercise.

And I did! I used the Aerobika twice a day, walked on the treadmill and went to Pilates classes, despite my embarrassing cough. Over the next six weeks, my cough let up and practically disappeared. It was just the boost I needed to stay motivated. Although my follow-up CT scan did not show any improvement, I felt better and more comfortable in social settings. When I was coughing non-stop, I had shied away from going to the movies, the theater and art lectures. All of these were things I loved. So, after once more enjoying my favorite activities, I was psyched to step up my self-care program.

When it comes to bronchiectasis, acceptance is crucial. What's done is done. Scarring is not going to disappear. Nevertheless, I knew I could create a healing environment in my body that would ward off harmful bacteria, soothe my airways and hopefully stop the scarring process. It was not just about doing; it was also about learning to let go and be patient. Being proactive with my bronchiectasis is at the core of who I am and how I handle life's challenges. At the same time, I knew I needed to relax to promote healing. As Glinda, the good witch in Oz said, "You've always had the power, my dear; you just had to learn it for yourself." So, I moved forward, trusting I would intuitively know when to act and when to be patient and rest.

I was warned not to take the content of Facebook support groups too much to heart. Many people who frequent such sites are quite ill and reach out to the group for comfort. Hospital stays, serious flare-ups, long courses of antibiotics and their side effects, and depression, are common topics in those online discussions. In spite of that warning, I felt a compulsive pull to the bronchiectasis community.

As predicted, while scrolling those sites, my anxiety would bubble up. It was paralyzing. My insides were being drenched in fight-or-flight hormones and chemicals; well-appreciated if you are being chased by a tiger... but not good for positive thinking. I believed I could keep my emotions in check and most of the time I did. These sites are a valuable source of information and camaraderie. Still, there were times when it was a challenge. Even the scholarly studies I read heightened my anxiety. In graduate school, I had done medical literature reviews and looked at findings objectively. Not so with my bronchiectasis. What I uncovered was extremely unsettling. Some of the Non-Cystic Fibrosis Bronchiectasis (NCFB) studies referenced mortality rates. I was puzzled because I had been told by trusted sources that people do not die from this disease; they die with it. So, why were researchers using death rates to determine the success of treatments? What I found was that a majority of the participants in these studies had severe bronchiectasis and frequent respiratory infections. Often bronchiectasis sufferers waited years, and in some cases, decades to be correctly diagnosed. By that time, many were not in the best condition to fight the disease. Furthermore, antibiotics were commonly used as a first measure and frequently people developed antibiotic-resistant infections.

Thankfully, health care providers have become increasingly aware of our disease. Moreover, the use of High-Resolution Computed Tomography (HRCT) scans to diagnose BE has become a game-changer in determining bronchiectasis today. What makes the treatment of bronchiectasis particularly challenging is that we are not a homogeneous group. Some of us have scarred airways from infections. Others have an underlying genetic, autoimmune or allergic condition with the result being bronchiectasis. Notwithstanding how we acquire bronchiectasis, one thing is certain—diagnosis of BE is on the rise. Bronchiectasis was once viewed as an orphan disease, a rare disease affecting fewer than 200,000 Americans. Recent studies show the prevalence of BE is much higher (Weycker et al., 2017).

Regardless of whether we have a mild or a more advanced case of bronchiectasis, whether we are currently taking medications or not, whether we have lots of energy or very little, self-care is critical. Self-care is not necessarily the easiest way to manage a disease, but it can be the most individualized, rewarding and hopefully successful way of living with a chronic condition.

The word "bronchiectasis" is a combination of the Greek words "bronckos" meaning airway and "ektasis" meaning widening or dilation. The last part, the "ektasis," makes it an irreversible disease as the tissue has lost its elasticity from inflammation and infection. Think of the stretched-out waistband of an old pair of pajama bottoms. No amount of laundering is going to shrink that band. The same is true of our lungs. However, self-care will make it easier to keep our overstretched passages from clogging with sticky mucus and organisms—bacteria, viruses and fungi—that cause infection and destroy tissue.

A crucial element of self-care is adopting a healthy lifestyle to decrease overall inflammation. A commitment to healthy eating, exercise and rest will make a significant difference. You must remain committed because your body is smart. It knows the difference between a few toe-touches and a one-hour exercise class. It knows the difference between shutting your eyes for five minutes and sitting down to your meditation practice fully present. It knows a quickie puff on an Aerobika versus a full-throttle attempt to get the mucus out.

Now let me be absolutely clear: **I am NOT advocating blowing off traditional medicine**. I am a firm believer in a healthcare team of conventional as well as alternative care providers. I also believe in taking advantage of every service your multi-disciplinary team of providers has to offer. I now have a care team that supports my healing and is available to answer questions as they arise. It took me some time and effort to get to this point, including traveling to another state for a second opinion and switching to a new pulmonologist who recommended that I see several other specialists to look for possible causes of my disease. Over time, I added in some complementary medical practitioners to help me heal. That way, I felt we were all working together and taking a holistic, individualized approach to my care. So, again, I urge those with BE to seek out the best medical care available in their community. If options are limited and you have the resources, find a top national specialist to guide your local team.

The BE CLEAR Method™ Philosophy

We are people with a life-long condition, but we are more than that condition. I will never refer to us as "patients." I am a person, not a patient. I have a full life that includes managing my condition, but I do not let bronchiectasis define me. My goal with this guide is just that—guidance. Some have the time, energy and the inclination to do it all. Others, especially those who are feeling poorly as well as those who work or have children at home, will most likely scale it back and concentrate on the essentials of exercise and airway clearance.

The BE CLEAR Method™ is a self-care framework for us to manage our disease. I am not a doctor, and I cannot give you medical advice. To that point, the method does not include any discussion of medications or supplements. All I can do is share with you my self-care exploration and tell you what I've found that works and does not work for me. Moreover, we are ever-changing beings on a physical, mental and spiritual level and are impacted by our environment and circumstances. What does not appeal to you at first might next month. Or what you do today might need to be modified in the future because of a health setback or life events. Being flexible is built into *The BE CLEAR Method to Living with Bronchiectasis*.

Also integral to BE CLEAR is making a promise to yourself that you will practice self-care daily. If you desire to improve your health, then you need to show up to do the work. Even if it means doing less than you usually do on a particular day, that is still something and it will keep you on track.

The best thing about managing your health is that you can test my suggestions and your modifications in the laboratory. The great news is that YOU are your own laboratory! If I recommend an exercise that I've found beneficial to do before airway clearance, you can test it out. For that matter, test it out in the morning, in the afternoon or before bed. Why? Because the lab is always open! Much of the mind/body work we do today was invented this way. Joseph Pilates is a perfect example. As a child in Germany, Joseph Pilates had asthma and other health issues. Motivated to overcome his physical challenges, he experimented and developed a comprehensive body wellness system.

So, why not you, too? In the BE CLEAR system I've outlined below, I have whittled down suggestions to only the easiest and most effective, but please experiment by modifying or enhancing as you see fit. Do what my favorite yoga teacher says and give yourself permission to "play with it." In other words, be creative, make it your own and do not take anything too seriously.

With that said, we have a serious disease that will be with us for life. But we can decide not to give it power over our spirit. As you go through the BE CLEAR approach, do not try to do everything at once, even if you are a proud overachiever. Furthermore, be kind to yourself and do not strive for perfection. Perfectionism and self-criticism are the antitheses of self-care. Okay then, are you ready to learn more about the BE CLEAR Method? Great, let's do it!

The BE CLEAR Method™

This self-care approach to living with bronchiectasis is called the BE CLEAR Method for two reasons. Firstly, as previously mentioned, BE is shorthand for bronchiectasis. Secondly, BE CLEAR is an acronym for the following:

- **B**reathing
- **E**xercise
- **C**learance of Airways
- **L**aughter
- **E**ating and Drinking
- **A**lternative Therapies
- **R**elaxation, Rest and Sleep

The BE CLEAR Method is a roadmap to feeling better with bronchiectasis, improving our health and preventing our condition from worsening. There is no cure for bronchiectasis, but if we diligently follow a self-care program based on the BE CLEAR Method, we can decrease the probability of flare-ups and exacerbations. Do not forget to get your doctor's approval of your plan. Many of us with bronchiectasis have other diseases, too. These comorbidities could preclude you from a few self-care options. Be cautious, start slowly and play with it!

The overarching concept of "being clear" means having:

- Clear lungs
- A mind clear of factual misconceptions about our disease
- A spirit that is clear of fear

Firstly, keeping our lungs clear is critical to living with bronchiectasis. If you get anything from this guide, it needs to be a daily commitment to removing mucus from airways through breathing, exercise and using clearance devices. This powerful trifecta is the key to a better quality of life. Whereas all three are important, I devote a lot of time to the

Exercise Chapter. I am passionate about exercise because it is the best way to clear our airways and realize other health benefits. So, no apologies for playing favorites!

Besides keeping our lungs clear, we can also benefit from clearing our minds of misconceptions about bronchiectasis. Anecdotes, like the ones posted on social media, are personal stories and may or may not be fact-based. If you go online to support others, that's great. If you go online to learn about BE, then scrutinize your sources. Online support forums are global, translating into a broad spectrum of therapies, outcomes and levels of patient education. For current information, you should visit the websites of top institutions and organizations that specialize in bronchiectasis. Throughout this guide, I cite reliable, evidence-based studies and references. Additional information can be found on my website *www.letsbecleartoday.com.*

Lastly, we must clear our thoughts of debilitating anger and fear. Maybe you were shocked by your diagnosis. I know I was. After a while, you might become resentful and perhaps angry about it. Perhaps that anger stems from your late diagnosis that resulted in unnecessary pulmonary scarring or that you now have to spend hours caring for yourself when you would rather be doing other things. Those in the advanced stages of this disease may be angry that their quality of life has diminished.

Negative emotions are expected, but over time, they will not serve us well. The hormones and other chemicals that are released in response to these emotions are harmful to our health. We will explore mindfulness and positive thinking in our chapters on "Laughter," "Alternative Therapies," and "Relaxation, Rest and Sleep." Suffice to say, if we are to achieve and maintain a nurturing environment in our bodies, one that is conducive to maximal healing and health, we need to clear negative thoughts quickly. So, smile. You're already on the right track.

Chapter 1

B is for Breathing

If you know the art of breathing you have the strength, wisdom, and courage of ten tigers.

CHINESE ADAGE

There is an endless number of therapeutic breathing techniques. While these breathing practices have various goals, the most imperative is to improve our diseased lungs' ability to oxygenate our bodies. This can give us more energy and reduce the probability of feeling short of breath and unwell.

The amazing fact is that we are always breathing without even thinking about it. Like blood circulation and digestion, our bodies are on auto-pilot when it comes to the intake of oxygen and the release of carbon dioxide, but breathing is in a class of its own. Even though breathing is automatic, unlike other bodily functions, we can consciously control our breathing. Studies show therapeutic breathwork can make a huge difference in oxygenating our bodies and reducing stress (Peterson, 2017). What initially feels forced eventually becomes second nature. Think of it as a new and improved auto-pilot. Most importantly, breathing practices can also help our bodies dislodge and clear mucus out of damaged airways, something I discuss in detail in the chapter on airway clearance.

BREATHING BEGINS WITH GOOD POSTURE

Before launching into breathing techniques and exercises, let's talk about posture. Posture is one of those topics no one wants to discuss. Maybe they find it dull, or maybe they find it difficult. But, for me, as a fitness and health educator, it is my favorite topic. Generally, I do not need to bring it up with clients, as they often broach the subject by commenting on my good posture. They ask me if I am a dancer, a huge compliment as I can barely follow the simplest dance moves! I explain that no, I am not a dancer, but at a young age my mother would say to me, "no one is pretty unless they stand up straight," and I took her words to heart.

Too often we go through life bent over like a question mark when we need to be more upright like an exclamation point. Sometimes our forward head position and rounded back are due to osteoporosis and other spinal changes that are not easily addressed. Be that as it may, changes can be made little by little over time. It all starts with wanting to straighten up and becoming hyper-vigilant about maintaining that pulled-up posture throughout the day until it becomes natural. But beware, there is a misconception about how to create good posture. You might have the urge to throw back your shoulders and lift up your chin. Stop! You will look like you are auditioning for a marching band and can end up with back pain!

Posture Exercise

Straightening out our spine and expanding our rib cage is integral to the BE CLEAR Method and it starts with mindfulness about our bodies in space. By following these simple instructions, you will considerably aid your lungs and diaphragm. Take a few minutes to check yourself out in a mirror. Is your head in front of your spine? Do you have a bit of an upper back hump? Are your arms rolling inward and palms facing back? What about the rest of your spine? We all have natural curves in our back that function as shock absorbers when we move, but are your curves particularly pronounced?

Now, pull up from the crown of your head, visualizing golden threads wrapping around the midday sun. Next, gently pull down from your tailbone while imagining roots growing into the earth. While holding this erect posture, relax your body so your stance is more natural, thereby allowing you to breathe deeply. Add movement to this exercise by taking ten steps and turning around and taking another ten steps. If you want a tactile cue, place a book on your head to keep the top of your head parallel with the ground. Over time you will notice a difference and see that without thinking about it, the way you carry yourself has improved. Remember to check in with your posture as you go about your day *especially* when sitting.

LINKING BETTER POSTURE TO BETTER BREATHING

Re-training our bodies after we have built up poor habits requires reminders and techniques. For example, when you catch yourself hunched over the computer, you can remind yourself, "sit up, breathe deeply." Or, you can even write it on a slip of paper and leave it on your desk. Over time, there will be less need to remind yourself to sit up and breathe. Your posture and deep breathing will be linked together as a new and healthy habit.

Do you think just sitting or standing straighter will automatically create better breathing without conscious effort? You could be right. Nonetheless, I bet there are impeccably postured ballerinas walking around my Lincoln Center neighborhood, home to the New York City Ballet, who would say they are shallow breathers. Reminding yourself to "stand straight, breathe deeply" will help create a new habit. Eventually, muscle memory will kick in and conscious effort will be minimally needed or not needed at all.

BREATHING TECHNIQUES AND PRACTICES

In this chapter, we discuss breathing techniques that can be used throughout the day. All of the practices I suggest combine slowing down and deepening the breath. Does it seem counterintuitive to slow down if our goal is to increase oxygen in our lungs? After all, won't taking more breaths bring in more air? Not necessarily. If we breathe quickly but not fully, sufficient air is not pulled down through our lungs to the alveoli, the berry-clustered breathing powerhouses at the ends of the lung branches. Quick, shallow ineffective breaths make the chest, shoulders, back and neck muscles work hard, causing us to feel fatigued instead of energized. Think about blowing up a balloon. Do twenty shallow breaths get the job done or would ten deep ones be better?

NASAL VERSUS MOUTH BREATHING

Many breathing techniques and theories address nose versus mouth breathing. Most certainly, if you go to yoga or meditation classes or do airway clearance, you have been told how to breathe. Frustratingly, you could have been given conflicting instructions. Here is what I think is best. As you go about your day, whenever possible, breathe in and out through your nose— because the nose is AWESOME. It sits prominently in the middle of your face seeking attention. Yet, rarely do we appreciate how efficiently and without complaint it accomplishes its long "to-do" list.

The nose is designed to stand guard and protect our bodies from harmful enemies. It does this through smell; a sniff test signals, for example, when leftovers need to be tossed. The nose also contains an army of little hairs, called cilia, that trap pathogens before they wreak havoc in our lungs. It further multi-tasks by swirling the air around in our nasal cavities, warming and moisturizing it before the journey into our lungs.

Understanding the nose's functions shows us how bypassing this port of entry by mouth-breathing is downright unfair to our bodies! We want our bodies to stay healthy and clear of disease, yet those of us who are mouth-breathers are rolling out the red carpet to pathogens and irritants. So, instead of breathing through your mouth and giving these bad dudes easy access to your lungs, make their journey difficult by, whenever possible, using your nose.

BELLY/DIAPHRAGMATIC BREATHING

"Belly breathing" is also referred to as "abdominal breathing" and "diaphragmatic breathing." But these terms are misleading, as our belly does not breathe and all breathing involves the diaphragm. The diaphragm is above our abdominal cavity and is the wizard behind the curtain. Over 20,000 times a day, it does its job of contracting downward with each inhalation to allow the chest to expand. Thank you diaphragm!

Our conventional way of thinking about inhaling is to suck in our gut, but this is not the way we enter the world and is certainly not the best way to breathe while we're in it. If you've ever observed babies breathe, you've seen their bellies puff up when inhaling. This action is what we are trying to recapture as it will lead to fuller breathing.

Belly Breathing Exercise

Lie on your back with your knees raised and your feet flat on the floor. Allow your knees to rest against one another. For extra comfort, you can put a thin pillow under your head. If you have gastric reflux (GERD), you might want to do this exercise on an empty stomach and with your head and chest elevated on pillows. With one hand on your belly and the other on your chest, inhale and exhale through your nose and observe how you currently breathe. Does your top hand (on your chest) move up and down with your breath more than your bottom hand (on your stomach)? How would you describe the quality of your breathing? Deep or shallow? Fluid or labored?

Now, move your hands to the sides of your ribcage. Any activity in the flanks? Do your ribs open up to assist the diaphragm in making room for lung activity? Or is there very little side expansion?

Belly breathing improves respiration by giving the lungs more space to expand. Use your abdomen pushing against your waistband as a tactile cue to deepen your breath by saying to yourself, "inhale deeply, belly expands." Now, to release the air, do nothing and it will happen naturally. Just put your attention on linking the inhalation with your belly expanding and allow your diaphragm to passively return during exhalation. If you find this exercise challenging, you can place something on your belly like a little pillow or a book to give you more tactile feedback. It is amazing how the physical and visual feedback of watching the object rise and fall can reinforce proper muscular engagement. Once you are comfortable doing this exercise lying down, try it without props and while sitting, then standing and finally while walking. Note any differences.

Not only do positions impact the ability to breathe deeply, so do activities such as eating and showering, talking on the phone, sitting at the computer, driving a car, climbing stairs and exercising. As you go through your day, observe your breath. You are probably not naturally belly breathing yet. Be patient. It will take time. With practice, muscle memory will kick in and your body will naturally switch to more belly breaths.

PURSED LIPS BREATHING

Earlier, I said to try and breathe in and out through your nose. However, when we are short of breath or have to calm ourselves, a technique called Pursed Lips Breathing (PLB) is most effective. With PLB we inhale through our nose and slowly and gently exhale through puckered lips as if cooling soup. This opens our airways and releases stale air trapped in our lungs. The slow exhalation allows the body to let go of tension.

Pursed Lips Breathing Exercise

The sensation of air flowing out against puckered lips is a perfect tactile cue. You can link this sensation to deep and steady breathing with the reminder "exhaling slowly against my lips allows a deep inhalation." Start practicing with three sets of five breaths and, when you are comfortable, increase the number of breaths. Be sure to sip water between sets.

BREATH COUNTING

In Belly Breathing the emphasis is on the inhalation, while in Pursed Lips Breathing, it is on the exhalation. With Breath Counting, it is on both; we lengthen the exhalation in relation to the inhalation. Some Breath Counting practices go back thousands of years to the ancient yogis while others are more contemporary. They vary in their ratio of inhalation to exhalation, for example, 1:2, 1:3, or 1:4. Although Breath Counting methods may differ, there is consensus on the benefit of the exhalation being longer than the inhalation.

Breath Counting Exercise

Do you know the ratio between your inhalation and exhalation? Check it out. Record the length of the inhalations and your exhalations and notice whether they are equal in length or if one is longer. Once you have an idea of how you usually breathe, extend the exhalations by one count. If, for example, you are at a ratio of two-count inhalations to three-count exhalations (2:3), extend the exhalations to four (2:4).

Likewise, if you are at three-count inhalations to four-count exhalations (3:4), aim for a 3:5 ratio. Challenge yourself, but do not strain. Let your body guide you.

BREATH COUNTING USING OVAL OF ENERGY IMAGERY

Unlike Diaphragmatic Breathing that causes the abdomen to rise, and Pursed Lips Breathing that we feel against our lips, Breath Counting does not have a handy visual or tactile cue. However, we can use imagery to keep our Breath Counting on track. My favorite is to picture my inhalation being pulled up my spine, starting at my tailbone and progressing up to the crown of my head. On my exhalation, I imagine a vibrant waterfall gushing down the front of my body. The imagery of "up-the-back, down-the-front" creates a continuous oval of energy and feels luxuriously supportive, even cocoon-like.

Breath Counting Using Oval of Energy Imagery Exercise

Inhale as you imagine your breath rising from your tailbone, up your back, to the top of your head. As you pull your inhalation up, say to yourself, "inhaling up 1,2,3." Once you reach the top, exhale your breath like a waterfall down the front of your body by saying to yourself, "exhaling down 1,2,3,4." Continue this dynamic oval of energy imagery for three rounds. Over time, add more breaths.

Alan Finger, co-founder of ISHTA Yoga, used this oval-waterfall imagery during a meditation class I took in 2003. It resonated with me and I continue to use it when consciously breathing and meditating. I recently heard Alexis Brink, head of the Jin Shin Institute in New York City, use similar imagery in her energy work. (I will discuss Jin Shin Jyutsu further in the Alternative Therapies Chapter.) For me, the egg-shaped oval has a regenerative, life-sustaining quality. It reminds me to inhale and take in nourishing breath, ideas and new experiences and to exhale and let go of what is no longer useful. In the following chapter on exercise, the breath continues to play a major role in bolstering our self-care efforts.

Bronchi-X-tra
Nasal Irrigation

Nasal irrigation (also called nasal lavage) is a practice that goes back to the ancient yogis. It is a method of rinsing out nasal passages to remove bacteria, viruses, fungi and irritants. It also hydrates the lining of the nasal cavity and reduces inflammation of the mucous membranes. Many people who have chronic pulmonary diseases regularly irrigate their nasal passages, even if they do not have sinus problems or upper respiratory infections. They maintain nasal hygiene as a safety measure to help keep their lungs clear.

This cleansing practice requires:

1. A neti pot or plastic squeeze bottle
2. Table salt or a commercially prepared mixture of sodium chloride and sodium bicarbonate
3. Previously boiled tap water or store-bought sterile water.

Once the salt and warm water are mixed, using a neti pot or squeeze bottle, the solution is slowly poured into one nostril with the head slightly tipped in the opposite direction. The solution will then run out from the other nostril. This process is repeated with the other nostril.

It is critical to follow instructions to keep your pot or bottle clean. I prefer to use a porcelain pot that can be sterilized in boiling water rather than a plastic bottle that cannot tolerate high heat.

Chapter 2

E is for Exercise

When it comes to health and well-being, regular exercise is about as close to a magic potion as you can get.

THICH NHAT HANH

Exercise impacts all bodily functions. It improves blood flow and respiration, aids digestion, strengthens muscles, calms nerves and reduces fatigue. Exercise can also lift one's mood, strengthen bones and prevent falls. In addition, for those with bronchiectasis, it can clear air passages of harmful mucus and reduce coughing. Dr. Noah Greenspan (2017) in his book *Ultimate Pulmonary Wellness,* says, "Exercise is by far, one of, if not *the* single best, most effective lifestyle change you can make and one of the most powerful tools to improve your health as well as your overall quality of life" (p.83). The European Respiratory Society (ERS) also stresses the importance of exercise. In their *Guidelines on the Management of Bronchiectasis*, they recommend that adults with BE exercise regularly (Chalmers et al., 2015). Likewise, the Chest Foundation, an American organization that champions lung health, states that exercise is one of the best ways to manage your health (Addrizzo-Harris et al., 2017, p.24).

Early on, when I was first diagnosed with BE, my understanding of the disease was limited. I thought my only symptom was my cough. Later, under the care of a new pulmonologist, I learned that the low-grade temperature and flu-ish feelings I occasionally experienced in the afternoons were also caused by bronchiectasis. For the most part, I only have these afternoon symptoms when I do not exercise to help clear my airways. It is a convincing reminder that, even with adequate sleep, eating right and using airway clearance devices, daily exercise is critical to my well-being.

THE NEED FOR DAILY EXERCISE TO CLEAR MUCUS OUT OF OUR LUNGS

If we were exercising strictly for strength or cardiovascular improvement, then doing so three or four times a week would be adequate. But we have the urgency of clearing our lungs to prevent further disease. Therefore, whenever possible, we need to exercise daily as part of our airway clearance regimen. (Airway clearance is the next chapter's topic.)

You can choose whether to exercise before or after using an airway clearance device. Test out what works best for you. Before you exercise, try using your Aerobika or a similar airway clearance device to remove irritating mucus and reduce coughing. Or, start your day with a morning workout to bring mucus up higher in your lungs and then use your clearance device. I will let you in on a little secret... sometimes I exercise while using my Aerobika! Back in the 80s there was a curly-haired art instructor on American television by the name of Bob Ross. He taught the ABCs of painting and would say things like, "Go ahead, add a little tree to your landscape. It's your world." How you choose to combine exercise with the use of a clearance device is the same—it's your world. Just know that doing both every day will make your world a better place.

BEGIN WHERE YOU ARE

For some, a busy work and family life will make daily exercise challenging. For others, physical and medical considerations such as joint pain, heart issues and fatigue might prevent them from feeling comfortable with exercise. And, frankly, for many, exercise is not something they ever wanted to do. With the BE symptoms of coughing, mucus production, exhaustion and, in some cases, urinary incontinence added to the mix, it is like asking them to climb Mount Everest!

In her book, *Start Where You Are*, Pema Chodron, a Buddhist nun, discusses the importance of starting any personal journey from wherever you are at that point in time. This concept can also be applied to how we think about exercise. Regardless of where we stand on the continuum, whether we are experienced or new to exercise, we can move forward slowly and carefully from our own unique place.

Being closely monitored and individually instructed at a pulmonary rehabilitation center is a great place to start if you are not already a regular exerciser. Then, on days when you do not go to rehab, you can follow an at-home program provided by the center or my Bronchi-X-ercise Strength, Stretch and Balance program (Bronchi-X-ercises for short) discussed in the following pages. An online pulmonary wellness program is also an option.

If you occasionally work out and are looking to increase the frequency and intensity of your exercise, then one-on-one sessions with an experienced certified personal trainer can put you on the right path. Even doing a couple of supervised workouts with a trainer and getting a tailor-made program you can do on your own is a great idea. Let your trainer know about your bronchiectasis and any other comorbidities you have and be sure to get medical clearance from your physician.

IT'S ALL ABOUT THE JOINTS

I often see people at the gym exercising with poor form. They launch into an exercise without taking time to set up correctly. For example, some use their body's momentum to swing weights with their arms… that is a great way to injure a shoulder joint! Others lift weights with rounded backs and no visible core engagement, thereby putting pressure on their spines. Granted, we do not need to be picture-perfect while exercising, but we do need to adhere to best practices while strength training to protect ourselves from injury. These practices begin with understanding what good postural alignment looks and feels like in our bodies so we can start each exercise from a safe position.

GOOD POSTURAL ALIGNMENT FOR EXERCISING AND LIVING

We all come in different packaging, but for the most part, healthy joint alignment means that when you look at your body side-on in a mirror you want to see soft, natural curves in your spine and:

- Your ear in a straight line above your shoulder
- Your shoulder in line with your hip
- Your hip in line with your knee
- Your knee in line with your ankle

When looking at your arms and legs while standing facing a mirror:

- The palms of your hands should face towards the side of your body not towards your back
- Your feet should point mostly forward

If you observe improper alignment, it might be due to one or more of the following:

- Sitting for hours a day with a rounded spine and forward head
- Sleeping propped up on extra pillows
- Coughing in a hunched position
- Weak muscles
- Tight muscles

CREATING MUSCLES THAT ARE TEAM PLAYERS

The body has over six hundred muscles that work together in complex ways. They all have jobs to do and work best when they are strong and lengthened. On the other hand, when muscles are tight and weak and not doing their fair share, they force other muscles to do double duty. So, we should strive to correctly utilize our muscles. It is like calling a sports huddle to encourage all players to do what they do best and work as a team. This way, our bodies will become more efficient, and hopefully, we will feel less tired.

The BE CLEAR Method includes a workout program called Bronchi-X-ercises. Based on traditional strength training and stretching techniques, this program goes further by including yoga and Pilates principles. Over time, Bronchi-X-ercises, or a similar program, can create a stronger and more flexible body. Bronchi-X-ercises can also help "X-out" mucus in the lungs and increase resilience to respiratory infections and flare-ups.

AEROBIC ACTIVITY AND THE BRONCHI-X-ERCISE STRENGTH, STRETCH AND BALANCE PROGRAM

According to the 2018 U.S. Health and Human Services Guidelines on exercise, adults with chronic conditions, if they are physically capable and have medical clearance, should try to do approximately 150 minutes of aerobic exercise weekly (Department of Health and Human Services [HHS], 2019, p.4). This equates to about twenty minutes of daily cardio activity. It can be any activity that gets your heart rate up such as walking, jogging, climbing stairs, biking, dancing or using cardio equipment.

Working up to a moderate effort is best: not too easy, not too hard. On a scale of 1-10, with one being super-easy and ten very vigorous, you should probably stay within a 3-4 moderate range unless your medical team recommends otherwise. If you are walking with someone, you should be able to talk, but your talking should be a bit labored (see the Bronchi-X-tra on Rate of Perceived Exertion and the Talk Test at the end of this chapter).

In time you may want to challenge yourself by adding thirty to sixty-second bursts of more vigorous activity. During these intervals your breathing will be more intense and you will not be able to talk comfortably. Always decrease your activity level at the end of your workout for approximately ten minutes to cool down.

If you enjoy keeping track of your progress with a device, you can use a heart rate monitor, a pedometer or an app on your phone. Otherwise, just enjoy your walk or bike ride. Consider challenging yourself when you feel ready by increasing the duration and/or difficulty of your exercise.

The U.S. federal guidelines on exercise for adults also recommend that weekly workouts include activities that strengthen muscles and improve balance (HHS, 2019). The Bronchi-X-ercise program consists of these elements as well as stretching. If you are new to exercise, familiarize yourself with the following terms:

> **Repetitions (reps)**—How many times you do an exercise. For example, 10 repetitions (reps) of leg lifts means lifting your leg 10 times.

> **Sets**— A group of consecutive reps. For example, 2 sets of 10 leg lifts mean 10 reps and then another 10 reps.

When you feel you can do both the Bronchi-X-ercises and the aerobic activity, experiment by doing them together and at separate times during the day. You can use the BE CLEAR Daily Exercise Checklist (at the end of the book) to keep a record. See what works best for you and switch it up from time to time.

SETTING UP FOR THE BRONCHI-X-ERCISE STRENGTH, STRETCH AND BALANCE PROGRAM

Bronchi-X-ercises are mindful movements coordinated with breathing. This means breathing steadily through each exercise to energize our bodies, focus our minds and get our internal fluids flowing. Exercises will include the following prompts unless otherwise indicated:

> **Set up** in the proper starting position as indicated on the exercise page.

Prepare by visualizing the exercise in the correct form and lengthening your spine. Drop your shoulders away from your ears, keep your neck and head in alignment with your spine, relax the back of your neck and your face and look straight ahead.

Inhale for the count of 2 while not moving (there are exceptions) to prepare to exercise.

Exhale with pursed lips (see the previous Breathing Chapter) for the count of 2 as you move per the exercise instructions. Continue using Pursed Lips Breathing as you repeat and/or hold the exercise. If you prefer, you can exhale through your nose.

Increase difficulty when you are ready by adding sets and/or using weights.

EXERCISE PRECAUTIONS

- *You should not experience pain while exercising.* If you have some mild muscle soreness a day or two after exercise, that is normal. Any persistent pain is not normal and you should seek medical care.
- When on your back, if you have a history of lower back discomfort, keep your legs bent.
- When on your back, if your head tilts back uncomfortably, place a thin pillow (about 3 inches high) or a folded towel under your head.
- Do not hold your breath. Generally, in the Bronchi-X-ercise program, you should inhale before lifting the weight, exhale with pursed lips as you lift it, and inhale as you return to your starting position. If this type of breathing is difficult for you, then just breathe normally.
- Use a neutral wrist when lifting weights. A neutral wrist means

your hand does not bend forward or backward at the wrist, but rather, it remains in line with your arm.

- When standing, press through your entire foot for maximum support. If you are on your hands and knees, spread your fingers.
- Exercise using good form. If you tire and begin to lose your ability to maintain good form, then eliminate or reduce the weight. Taking a break to breathe slowly and deeply might also recharge you.
- Some exercises call for a standing position but if this is difficult for you, then sit. Many Bronchi-X-ercises can be done in either position. If the exercise does not work for you sitting, then skip the exercise and go on to the next one.
- If it is difficult for you to get down to and up from the floor, use a bed. For additional firmness, use a firm exercise mat on the bed.
- If you have gastric reflux (GERD), consult your doctor before performing any exercises on your back and/or any exercise that positions your hips higher than your head. Basic precautions for GERD include:

  ◊ Waiting a couple of hours after eating before exercising.
  ◊ Doing exercises while standing or sitting, whenever possible.
  ◊ When on your back, elevating your head and chest with pillows so that your upper body is at a 30-degree angle.

EXERCISING EQUIPMENT FOR HOME WORKOUTS

- 2 or 3-pound weights
- 1-2 pound ankle weights
- 6 feet of green Theraband. Therabands are color-coded to indicate their level of resistance. Green is moderate. If you have never exercised, use red or yellow. If green is too easy, use blue.
- A non-slip exercise mat

JUICING THE JOINTS WARM-UP

Juicing the Joints gently wakes up the body and coats the joints with protective synovial fluid. Just like coating a baking pan with oil when making a cake, we should take similar precautions when exercising. There are endless choices for going about this, yet it can be as simple as putting on music and dancing around! Whether you are doing the Mashed Potato to James Brown or the Swim to the Beach Boys, use both your arms and legs and make your movements gentle. A ten-minute ride on an exercise bike or a walk on a treadmill is also a good choice.

People who do not have the energy to stand can dance from a seated position. When you feel better then by all means take your moves to the dance floor! But, until then, clockwise and counterclockwise arm circles and marching knee lifts should sufficiently lubricate your joints. If you are very fatigued, you may choose to just do Juicing the Joints movements as your daily workout until you can add more specific exercises into the mix.

Now that you are warmed up, let's bronchi-X-ercise! There are ten exercises in the program. Try to do them in the order listed in the chart. See how the Bronchi-X-ercises feel and if any of them are too difficult or uncomfortable, skip them, do fewer repetitions, use lighter weights or eliminate weights altogether. Perform these exercises three or four times a week or whatever feels right for you.

The Bronchi-X-ercise Strength, Stretch and Balance Program

	NAME	POSITION	PURPOSE	TO INCREASE DIFFICULTY	OPTIONAL ACCESSORY	REPS/ HOLD
1	Wall Push Up	Standing	Muscle Integration + Strength + Stretch			10 reps
2	Front and Back Leg Lift	Standing	Strength + Balance	Ankle weights, not holding on to support	Ankle weights	10 reps per each exercise
3	Heel Raise and Balance	Standing	Strength + Balance	Ankle weights, not holding on to support, longer hold on toes	Ankle weights	10 reps with count of 1 when holding on toes
4	Shoulder Blade Squeeze with Band	Sitting	Strength + Stretch	Heavier band		10 reps
5	"V" Arm Raise with Band	Sitting	Strength	Heavier band or hand weights	Hand weights instead of band	10 reps
6	Chest Fly with Weights	On Back	Strength	Heavier hand weights	Pillow for GERD	10 reps
7	Bent Leg Marching	On Back	Strength	Ankle weights	Ankle Weights, Pillow for GERD	10 reps
8	Hamstring and Calf Stretch with Band	On Back	Stretch		Pillow for GERD	Count of 30 hold
9	Belly Draw-In	On Hands and Knees	Strength			5 reps
10	Pointer Dog	On Hands and Knees	Integration + Strength + Stretch + Balance	Opposite arm and leg lift, count of 10, with hand and ankle weights	Hand weights, Ankle weights	5 reps holding each for count of 5

1.Wall Push Up

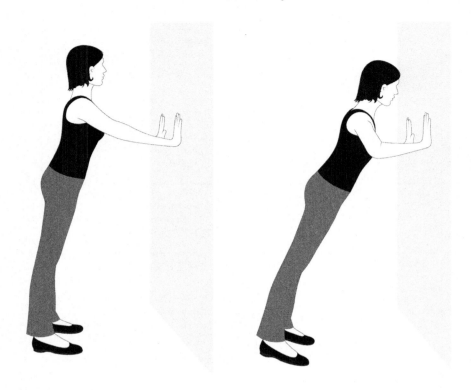

Set-up: Stand with your feet hip-width apart and face a wall at approximately an arm's length distance.

Place your hands on the wall (a little wider than your shoulders and a little lower than shoulder height). You should be comfortable. If not, adjust yourself accordingly. Position your feet facing forward to the best of your ability.

Prepare: Take a few breaths as you visualize this exercise. Lengthen your spine. Drop your shoulders. Relax the back of your neck and your face.

Inhale for a count of 2 as you bend your elbows. Keep your body in a straight line. Resist the tendency to move your head forward and out of alignment with your body.

Exhale through pursed lips for a count of 2 as you straighten your arms (with a slight bend at the elbow) to return to your starting position.

Perform 10 repetitions. Add a second set when you are stronger.

2. Front and Back Leg Lift

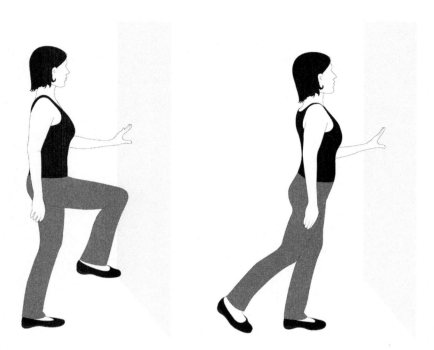

Set-up: Stand with your feet hip-width apart and facing a wall with enough room to be able to raise your bent leg (Front Leg Lift can also be done seated).

Lightly hold on to the wall for support. This exercise can also be done holding on to a counter or chair. Position your feet facing forward to the best of your ability.

Prepare: Take a few breaths as you visualize this exercise. Lengthen your spine. Drop your shoulders. Relax the back of your neck and your face.

Inhale for a count of 2 without moving.

Exhale through pursed lips for a count of 2 as you raise your bent right leg until your thigh is parallel with the floor or lower if this is too difficult.

Inhale for a count of 2 as you return your leg to the starting position.

Perform 10 repetitions and then repeat on the left side.

Next, do another set of 10, but this time bring your leg behind you. Remain upright without tilting forward.

Add a second set when you are stronger. Increase difficulty by lessening hold or not holding support and adding ankle weights.

3. Heel Raise and Balance

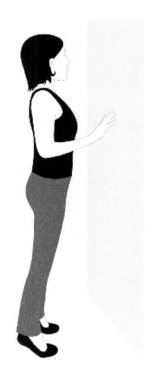

Set-Up: Stand with your feet hip-width apart and facing a wall.

Lightly hold on to the wall for support. This exercise can also be done holding on to a counter or chair.

Position your feet facing forward to the best of your ability.

Prepare: Take a few breaths as you visualize this exercise. Lengthen your spine. Drop your shoulders. Relax the back of your neck and your face.

Inhale for a count of 2 without moving.

Exhale through pursed lips for a count of 2 as you rise up onto your toes and balance for a count of 1.

Inhale for a count of 2 as you lower your heels back to the floor.

Perform 10 repetitions.

Add a second set when you are stronger. Increase difficulty by holding for a count of 2 while on your toes, lessening hold or not holding support and adding ankle weights.

4. Shoulder Blade Squeeze with Band

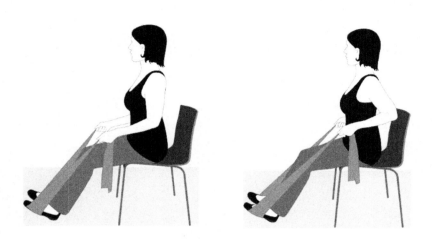

Set-Up: Sit in a chair with both legs slightly bent and extended comfortably in front of you.

Position the band securely beneath the middle of your feet as shown in the picture. With bent arms, grasp the ends of the band with a little tension in the band. Use a neutral wrist as previously described.

Prepare: Take a few breaths as you visualize this exercise. Lengthen your spine. Drop your shoulders. Relax the back of your neck and your face.

Inhale for a count of 2 without moving.

Exhale through pursed lips for a count of 2 as you squeeze your shoulder blades together and pull the band so that your elbows bend and go behind your torso. Imagine squeezing a long balloon between your shoulder blades. Adjust the length of the band so that the exercise is challenging but not too difficult.

Inhale for a count of 2 as you return to your starting position.

Perform 10 repetitions. Add a second set when you are stronger and/or use a heavier band.

5. "V" Arm Raise with Band

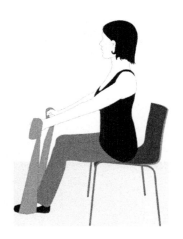 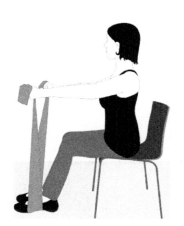

Set-Up: Sit in a chair with both legs bent and extended comfortably in front of you.

Position the band securely beneath the middle of your feet.

With arms extended with a slight bend at the elbow, grasp the ends of the band with some tension in the band. Use a neutral wrist as previously described. You may use weights instead of the band.

Prepare: Take a few breaths as you visualize this exercise. Lengthen your spine. Drop your shoulders. Relax the back of your neck and your face.

Inhale for a count of 2 without moving.

Exhale through pursed lips for a count of 2 as you raise your arms in front of you, at shoulder height in a "V." Engage your belly muscles and try not rock backward.

Adjust the length of the band so that the exercise is challenging but not too difficult. You can use hand weights instead of the band if you prefer.

Inhale for a count of 2 as you return to your starting position.

Perform 10 repetitions.

Add a second set when you are stronger and/or use a heavier band or weights.

6. Chest Fly with Weights

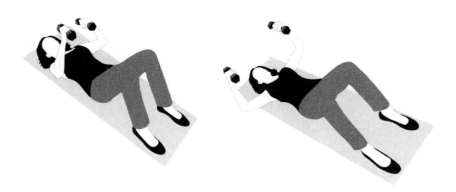

Set-Up: Lie on your back with legs bent, in line with your hips and with your feet on the floor. Place pillows under your head and chest if you have GERD and wish to make this adjustment.

Position your feet facing forward to the best of your ability.

Hold weights and extend arms in front and above your chest with arms bent and hands about 5 inches apart (as if hugging a tree).

Prepare: Take a few breaths as you visualize this exercise. Lengthen your spine. Drop your shoulders. Relax the back of your neck and your face. Lightly pull in your lower abs as you gently press your back against the floor or pillow.

Inhale for a count of 2 as you open your arms while maintaining bent elbows. Take care not to arch your back.

Exhale through pursed lips for a count of 2 as you return to your starting position.

Perform 10 repetitions.

Add a second set when you are stronger and/or use heavier weights.

7. Bent Leg Marching

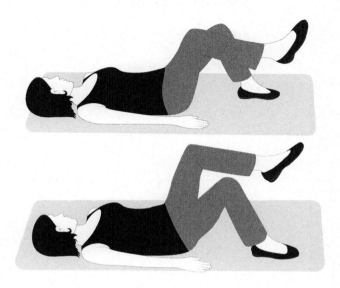

Set-Up: Lie on your back with legs bent, hip-width apart and feet on the floor. Place pillows under your head and chest if you have GERD and wish to make this adjustment.

Position your feet facing forward to the best of your ability.

Arms at your side.

Prepare: Take a few breaths as you visualize this exercise. Lengthen your spine. Drop your shoulders. Relax the back of your neck and your face. Lightly pull in your lower abs as you gently press your back against the floor or pillow.

Inhale for a count of 2 without moving.

Exhale through pursed lips for a count of 2 as you lift your right foot 12 inches off the floor. Keep your tailbone on the mat.

Inhale for a count of 2 as you return to your starting position.

Exhale through pursed lips for a count of 2 as you lift your left foot 12 inches off the floor.

Inhale for a count of 2 as you return to your starting position.

Perform 10 repetitions, alternating between your right and left leg. The combination of a right and left foot lift counts as 1 rep.

Add a second set when you are stronger. Increase difficulty by touching the floor with just your toes and/or adding ankle weights.

8. Hamstring and Calf Stretch with Band

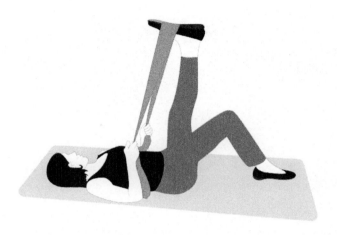

Set-Up: Lie on your back with legs bent, hip-width apart and feet on the floor. Place pillows under your head and chest if you have GERD and wish to make this adjustment.

Position the band under your right foot while your leg is still bent. Hold the ends of the band with both hands, arms at your side.

Prepare: Take a few breaths as you visualize this exercise. Lengthen your spine. Drop your shoulders. Relax the back of your neck and your face. Lightly pull in your lower abs as you gently press your back against the floor or pillow.

Inhale for a count of 2 without moving.

Exhale through pursed lips for a count of 2 as you straighten and raise your leg. It does not need to straighten completely or come to a 90-degree angle. Find the place where you feel a stretch. Now hold it there for a count of 30 while you inhale and exhale. Do not hold your breath.

Gently return your foot to the floor and repeat on the left side.

9. Belly Draw-in

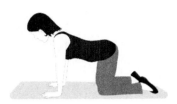 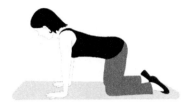

Set-Up: On your hands and knees. Your hands should be directly under your shoulders and your knees directly under your hips.

Allow your belly to soften and hang low. Keep your spine level with the floor, not letting it sag or round during this exercise.

Prepare: Take a few breaths as you visualize this exercise. Lengthen your spine. Relax your shoulders, the back of your neck and your face. Keep your head in alignment with your spine. Do not allow your head to hang down.

Inhale for a count of 2 without moving.

Exhale through pursed lips for a count of 5 as you draw in your abdominal muscles towards your spine while maintaining a flat back. Do not round your back.

Inhale for a count of 2 as you relax your belly and return to your starting position.

Perform 5 repetitions.

Add a second set when you are stronger.

10. Pointer Dog

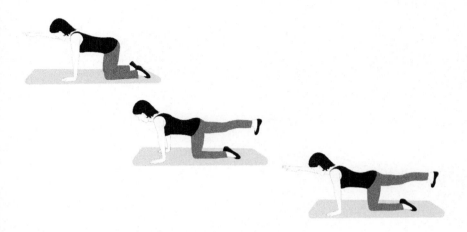

Set-Up: On your hands and knees. Your hands should be directly under your shoulders and your knees directly under your hips. Spread your fingers to increase stability.

Prepare: Take a few breaths as you visualize this exercise. Relax your shoulders, the back of your neck and your face. Keep your head aligned with your spine. Do not look up or allow your head to hang down.

Inhale for a count of 2 without moving.

Exhale through pursed lips for a count of 5 as you lift your right hand off the mat. Stretch your arm straight out in front of you and parallel to the floor. Do not hold your breath.

Inhale for a count of 2 as you return to your starting position.

Exhale for a count of 5 as you lift your left hand off the mat. Stretch your arm straight out in front of you and parallel to the floor. Do not hold your breath.

Inhale for a count of 2 as you return to your starting position.

Perform 5 repetitions. The combination of right and left counts as 1 rep. Add a second set when you are stronger. Repeat using only your legs.

Increase difficulty by extending opposite arms and legs simultaneously. Do not hold your breath.

HITTING THE GYM--HOW TO HANDLE COUGHING OR THE FEAR OF COUGHING IN EXERCISE CLASS

Mucus production, coughing and throat clearing are embarrassing and can stop some of us from participating in exercise classes. I, too, have experienced the embarrassment of coughing and having to assure fellow class participants that I am not contagious. I have also found myself shying away from going to classes out of fear of coughing. No two ways about it, coughing or the fear of coughing can be an exercise buzzkill. I have several ways of dealing with these concerns that I think you will find helpful:

- Clear your airways before going to class.
- Sip water during class to clear mucus from the back of your throat.
- Attend classes with music that will make your coughing less noticeable.
- Choose classes that begin with you standing rather than lying down.
- Vary your classes so you are not always with the same people.
- Vary where you position yourself in class so you do not feel that you are constantly disturbing the same people.
- If you prefer to go to the same class and occupy the same place in the room, make friends with those around you and let them know your cough is not contagious.
- Stay in the back of the class in case you start coughing and want to temporarily leave the room.
- Be a little selfish and think of the class as what you need to do to stay healthy and try not to obsess if you cough.
- Do not forget to breathe deeply to remain calm and enjoy yourself.

A SPECIAL NOTE TO THOSE WHO FEEL THEY ARE TOO UNWELL TO EXERCISE

Please do not despair! This chapter might seem like I am asking you to do the impossible. Here is my suggestion: pick a couple of exercises that look doable. For example, wall push-ups can be done without fully bending your arms... then why not throw in some heel raises while you're at it? What about some of the exercises and stretches that you can do in bed? Start with one set (5 repetitions of each exercise might be enough) and over time add more reps, more sets or even new exercises. Lastly, if "exercise" is still an unpleasant thought, think of it as movement. Strengthening your body through movement can make it easier for you to do practical things like making your bed, drying your hair and the topic of the next chapter, clearing your airways.

REGULAR EXERCISERS SHOULD BE VIGILANT

Those of you who exercise at a high intensity should monitor yourselves. If you are wrung out, have a lot of mucus or develop a low-grade temperature, you might want to take your exercise down a notch. Now in my 60s, I find that when my activity is too strenuous, I sometimes feel unwell later in the day. Rather than risk it, I do a morning and late afternoon workout at a moderate intensity. We are all different and the best approach is to be mindful and honest with how we feel. Our goal is to exercise to get stronger and clear our airways, not to cause additional inflammation.

Bronchi-X-tra
Rate of Perceived Exertion (RPE)
Talk Test

Rate of Perceived Exertion (RPE) is a self-determined evaluation of your level of physical effort while exercising. Although there are different systems with their own number ranges, I like to use the 0-10 rating. When we determine our RPE while exercising, we take into account muscle weariness and discomfort, how hard we are breathing and even our psychological state. RPE is a good way to check in with ourselves to see if we are exercising at the proper level. Moderate exercise would be rated a 3, heavy exercise a 5 and very heavy exercise a 7. The Cleveland Clinic suggests a rating of 3-4 in most cases, but be sure to adhere to whatever your medical team recommends.

The **Talk Test** is another easy way to measure the intensity of exercise. If you can talk with a minimum of difficulty while exercising, it is considered moderate effort. If, for example, you are walking about three miles an hour or bicycling about ten miles per hour on relatively flat terrain, you would probably be in the moderate zone. However, if you are ramping it up with activities like jogging, uphill walking or jumping rope, you would most likely be unable to say more than a few words at a time. You would therefore be working at a vigorous intensity. Exercising alone? Try reciting your favorite poem or counting to twenty out loud to gauge your exercise intensity.

Chapter 3

C is for Clearance of Airways

You always have two choices: your commitment versus your fear.

SAMMY DAVIS JR

Those of us with bronchiectasis have areas of flabby, stretched-out airway passages that collect mucus. To stay our healthiest, we must set aside time each day to clear out mucus that has accumulated in those areas. Unlike exercise that can often be enjoyable, such as walking with a friend, playing tennis or dancing to a favorite song, there is nothing pleasurable about twenty to forty minutes spent trying to expectorate mucus! Sure, we can put on a movie or binge-watch a TV show, but this solitary activity requires focus and effort. Also, I'll just come out and say it… having to cough up this gunk from our lungs is gross!

You might think it is unprofessional to say mucus is disgusting, but we are just people who are trying to care for ourselves, not respiratory therapists doing a job. This is our daily reality and it is not a fun activity. It is also a noisy process that involves lots of coughing and huffing and puffing. It often makes me feel like the wolf in the Three Little Pigs, trying to blow the house down. It may be melodramatic, but I want to go on record saying I do not like daily airway clearance. Yet, I know it is critical to prevent exacerbations and bronchiectasis progression.

With this urgency in mind, I have embraced daily clearance and if you are not currently doing it every day, I hope I can convince you to start. According to Registered Respiratory Therapist Cheryl Torres, people should not get discouraged if they do not bring up mucus when they do their clearance. Often the action is happening "behind the scenes," and patients will benefit from practicing daily clearance (personal communication, February 20, 2021).

In healthy lungs, many microscopic hairs called cilia work in a synchronized way to sweep out gunk from air passages. However, in damaged lungs, there are areas where cilia have been destroyed. Without an entire army of these little sweepers to keep our lungs clean, harmful bacteria and other organisms can pool in dilated, ineffective airways. For this reason, we must use Airway Clearance Techniques (ACTs) to move mucus, dirt and debris along and prevent the harmful inflammation and infection that characterize the progression of bronchiectasis.

In Facebook bronchiectasis support groups, I see many who do not perform daily airway clearance because they are not bothered by mucus or a persistent cough. I was of the same mindset until I had a bronchoscopy, a procedure whereby a tiny camera is inserted into the lungs so your doctor can look around and collect samples for laboratory analysis. I went into the procedure assuming that since I was no longer coughing, my lungs were relatively clear. I was shocked to later read the lab report describing "copious mucopurulent secretions" and "mucus plugs." It was a good lesson that the absence of a cough and mucus does not necessarily mean that there is not bad stuff in there. This is why airway clearance needs to be done every day and not just when we get sick.

As of the beginning of 2021, the United States does not have guidelines for the management of bronchiectasis. However, several countries and organizations including the British Thoracic Society have published guidelines and all acknowledge the importance of airway clearance (Hill et al., 2019). Dr. Pamela McShane, a leading pulmonologist in infectious lung disease, gives a compelling reason for daily airway clearance by comparing it to flossing. We floss daily to disturb biofilm between our teeth (a practice many do even with no apparent food bits to remove). Likewise, breaking up bacteria biofilm in our lungs should be our motivation for airway clearance (NTM Info & Research, 2020).

Keeping our lungs clear of mucus is not a new concept. Over 200 years ago, René Laennec, a French physician and the inventor of the stethoscope, first identified bronchiectasis as "the long continuance of… voluminous sputum." Laennec further stated, "… it is evident that the only means we possess of restoring the bronchi to their natural size is by diminishing the secretion of the mucous membrane." (Chalmers & Sibila, 2020) After two centuries of experience with bronchiectasis, we know that although there is no way for adults with BE to return stretched-out airways to their natural size, we do need to keep them clear. In their article *Happy Birthday, Bronchiectasis: 200 Years of Targeting Mucus*, Chalmers and Sibila say researchers need a better understanding of the properties of mucus and the most effective ways to reduce accumulation in the airways.

MY EXPERIENCE WITH AIRWAY CLEARANCE

Your medical team will choose the right airway clearance for you, factoring in the location of bronchiectasis in your lungs and the disease's progression. However, I have often heard that the best method of clearing airways is the one you are willing and able to do regularly. This activity is usually done once or twice a day and even more frequently during respiratory infections and flare-ups. Hopefully, you will be able to meet with a therapist to review airway clearance. I say hopefully because, even in New York City, I had difficulty finding a therapist with this expertise. When I asked my first pulmonologist to refer me to a therapist specializing in airway clearance, he said he did not know anyone! Instead, I had a ten-minute clearance session with his nurse who asked me to choose between an Acapella® and an Aerobika®.

I knew nothing about these devices so I blindly chose the Aerobika. Four months later when I attended a New York City support group, I learned that although most used the Aerobika some preferred the Acapella, so I bought one, too. After experimenting, I still prefer the Aerobika but occasionally switch things up with the Acapella. There are a few considerations for using these devices, so it is prudent to get your health professional's approval before ordering one online.

I was not comfortable with the limited patient education I received in my doctor's office, so I searched online for other resources. I found the Pulmonary Wellness & Rehabilitation Center in New York City and met with a therapist to review my airway clearance. Even though the center was not on my health plan, I felt it was key for an experienced therapist to teach me the best ways to clear my airways; something I have come to see as both a science and an art. A year later when I switched to a new pulmonologist, she referred me to an in-house hospital therapist. I had several visits with the therapist who evaluated my clearance techniques and made some recommendations. At a couple of our sessions, he percussed me like a bongo drum. His technique did not produce more sputum than what I did at home and it felt empowering to know that I was doing a good job on my own.

AIRWAY CLEARANCE TECHNIQUES (ACTS)

Below are some Airway Clearance Techniques (ACTs) including breathing practices, clearance devices and oscillating vests. I cover these ACTs with a brief description for each of them. This way, you will know about these options and can discuss them with your care team. Although I mention that I nebulize sodium chloride, I will leave the discussion of mucus thinning medications as well as bronchodilators, inhaled corticosteroids and antibiotics to medical professionals.

As you clock in airway clearance hours, trying new approaches and getting input from your therapist along the way, you will learn which clearance tools in your bronchiectasis toolbox work best for you and when to use them. There is an expression, "A new broom sweeps the floor, but an old broom knows the corners." I hope once you get adequate professional input and try different practices, you will have the experience to know how to "sweep your corners" and have clearer lungs.

BREATHING TECHNIQUES

Breathing methods such as **Active Cycle Breathing Therapy** (ACBT) and **Autogenic Drainage** (AD) are the oldest and most researched airway clearance techniques. Therapists throughout the world use them to treat bronchiectasis and teach them to patients to do at home. These breathing methods use various breathing styles with the mainstays being relaxed breathing, deep breathing and huffing. The goal is to keep the airways open with your breath to allow the mucus to come loose, then move it up to the point where you can cough or huff-cough it out.

I often use the huff-cough (exhaling as if fogging a mirror) instead of a more forceful cough because I am mildly hoarse and it is gentler on my vocal cords. During huffing, the vocal cords stay open and allow mucus to exit the lungs unimpeded. I think of it as trying to let a moth out of the house. The moth can more easily escape when you hold the door open. That is what you are doing while huffing.

If your health team has not suggested breathing practices as part of your daily clearance, you can look on YouTube for ones to try. You will notice slight differences in how the techniques are performed but do not let that throw you. Choose which ones you want to experiment with, get your team's approval, and then practice daily. You may have gathered from the chapter on breathing that while breathing techniques may seem simple, they are deceptively tricky because when we are no longer working with a therapist and are on our own, we have to work hard to stay focused. It is not an exaggeration to say that in this world of multitasking, endless to-do lists and distractions galore, dedicating two sessions a day to breathing can be daunting.

I use various breathing practices, along with my clearance devices, which are discussed below. I feel less pressure to get my breathing precisely right when I know my device will help me get the job done. This relaxes me, which I find to be the most important factor in my airway clearance. If I am stressed or hurried and trying too hard to clear my lungs, then little if anything happens. The relaxed and deep breathing between rounds with the Aerobika prevents me from breathing too forcefully into the device, potentially collapsing my airway passages and trapping mucus. Also, practically speaking, there will be times when you are away from home without your clearance device and feel mucus accumulating in the back of your throat. Knowing how to use your breath to remove bothersome secretions until you return home for a more thorough clearance is invaluable.

OSCILLATING POSITIVE EXPIRATORY PRESSURE THERAPY

The Aerobika® and the Acapella®

Oscillating Positive Expiratory Pressure (OPEP), a technology used in devices such as the Aerobika® and the Acapella®, is a game-changer in airway clearance. These airway clearance instruments are lightweight, easy to use, effective at moving out mucus and small enough to pop into your bag. Furthermore, since we are used to holding our phones 24/7, having a hand-held airway clearance gizmo is familiar and gives our practice that state-of-the-art feeling. For me, this user-friendly invention is akin to the latest iPhone.

The Aerobika and Acapella work with your exhalation to open your airways and unstick the mucus from weak and collapsed airway walls. Additionally, these OPEP devices make mucus less sticky. A distributor of the Aerobika describes the medical technology as having a "frequency range of… oscillations (that) corresponds with the natural process of the cilia, helping move mucus to the larger airways of the lungs where it can be coughed out." (Monaghanmed, n.d.) The Aerobika earned international recognition as a top medical innovation that improves the quality of life and patient care. I like the device's design as it looks like a rescue inhaler so when I use it in public, I do not feel conspicuous.

Both the Aerobika and Acapella can be used either sitting up or lying down and both devices allow the user to set the amount of resistance against their exhalation. Also, both can accommodate attaching a nebulizer. A nebulizer is a separate device that turns liquid medication into a mist that is then inhaled into the lungs. Many people save time with their clearance program by attaching the nebulizer to their OPEP device rather than using them separately. I use them together when time is an issue, but I prefer to use them separately. When I use them attached, the process goes by so quickly that my body doesn't have time to relax and let go.

Furthermore, if the nebulizer with its liquid medication is attached to the Aerobika, lying on my back or side can cause the liquid to drip out. That is why I often first nebulize sitting up and then use just the Aerobika in various postural positions that use gravity to help my lungs drain. Keep in mind that if you have gastric reflux (GERD), postural drainage might not be a good option for you or you might need to wait several hours after eating before lying down.

LUNG FLUTE®

The Lung Flute® is another hand-held device that differs from the Aerobika and Acapella by using low-frequency acoustic waves to break up mucus. As you exhale into the long tube forcefully enough to make the reed oscillate, the sound waves go deep into the lungs and break up mucus. At the Pulmonary Wellness & Rehabilitation Center, my therapist recommended I try using the Flute in the morning to see if it was more effective than the Aerobika in clearing deeper secretions. I did not notice any benefit over the Aerobika and found the larger-size Flute more cumbersome and harder to sterilize. Even so, I like having it as another tool in my BE toolbox and use it now and then, especially if I am not able to cough out much with my other clearance techniques.

HFCWO VESTS

Many in the U.S. bronchiectasis community use High-Frequency Chest Wall Oscillation (HFCWO) vests. There are several manufacturers of these vests, and they vary in their technology, portability and comfort. They work by vibrating and putting pressure on the rib cage to move secretions in the lungs. Most people wear them daily while they nebulize and use their OPEP device. HFCWO vests are expensive, but insurance companies in the United States generally cover them with a bronchiectasis diagnosis. Recently my doctor suggested that I try a vest and I am hopeful that it will make a difference with my airway clearance.

For all the good work these devices can do, let's not forget that exercise plays an important role in clearance, too. In fact, all current bronchiectasis guidelines recommend that exercise be part of airway clearance regimens. Those who cannot tolerate much exercise will mainly rely on breathing therapies and devices; however, over time and with professional guidance, I hope you can add in daily movement and stretching to open your chest. It could start with simple arm swings and other "Juicing the Joints" movements. Eventually, as you begin to better tolerate a broader range of motion and movement, it could lead to more movement intensity, cleaner lungs, better breathing and a higher quality of life.

It is time to stop thinking about all these "should-dos" that require a daily commitment. Yes, we all know to take it day by day, but at the same time, the thought of doing all this huffing and puffing is tiring and, for some, depressing. So, let's take a few deep breaths, pour ourselves a tall glass of water and get comfy. The next chapter of the BE CLEAR Method is on laughter. As the comedian Milton Berle said, "laughter is an instant vacation" and by now, we could all use one!

Chapter 4

L is for Laughter

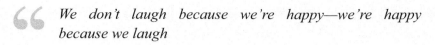

We don't laugh because we're happy—we're happy because we laugh

WILLIAM JAMES

KNOCK, KNOCK!
Who's there?
Banana.
Banana who?
Knock, knock.
Who's there?
Banana.
Banana who?
Knock, knock.
Who's there?
Orange.
Orange who?
Orange you glad I didn't say banana?

You may not find this joke particularly funny, unlike my young grandsons who think it is hysterical. No matter how many times they tell it, it sends them into a fit of giggles. Then, their laughter becomes contagious and before long I am laughing along with them.

The adage "laughter is the best medicine" was verified by Norman Cousins, editor of the *Saturday Review,* in his groundbreaking book *Anatomy of an Illness* published in 1979. The book details his painful experience with a degenerative disease. When Cousins was told there was only a one in 500 chance of going into remission, he took matters into his own hands by creating a laughter therapy program for himself. He found that laughing at comedy shows like Candid Camera, The Three Stooges and The Marx Brothers eased his pain and was a large part of his recovery. Although many in the medical community were skeptical of his claims, Cousins said, "We mustn't regard any of this as a substitute for competent medical attention. But the doctor can only do half the job. The other half is the patient's response to the illness. What we really mean by a patient's responsibility is that we've got vast powers that are rarely used. It's important to avoid defeatism and a sense of panic and despair." (Colburn, 1986)

Surprisingly, the New England Journal of Medicine published Cousins' article about his layman's approach and self-experimentation. His publication made the medical profession sit up and pay attention. Although many physicians had doubts about Cousins' unscientific approach, he had laid down the gauntlet. Several researchers in the 1980s took up the challenge, including Dr. Lee Berk, a preventive care specialist in California. Berk and his colleagues conducted many experiments involving laughter. In one study, they measured the participants' stress hormones before and after watching an hour of comedy. After watching the show, the study found the subjects had lower stress hormones than those who did not watch it (Berk et al., 1989).

Laughter is also known to increase the hunger hormone ghrelin. As Berk explains, repetitive laughter causes ghrelin to rise, similar to the effects exercise has on increasing appetite (Federation of American Societies for Experimental Biology [FASEB], 2010). This is noteworthy for those who have lost their appetite from the side effects of medications and bouts of depression (which often occurs with bronchiectasis). Research shows that individuals with bronchiectasis who stay within a normal weight range fare better than those who are underweight (Qi, 2015).

In 1995, Dr. Matan Kataria, an Indian physician living in Mumbai, started a laughing club. The club's formation was based on research by Dr. Kataria on the health benefits of laughter. His concept caught on and was called "Hasya Yoga" which means "Laughter Yoga." Today, there are thousands of Laughter Yoga Clubs throughout the world. Several years ago while on vacation, I went to a Laughter Yoga class. I hemmed and hawed about going to the class thinking it sounded silly, but eventually I gave in. Following the teacher's instructions, our group of about twenty women formed a circle and did some deep breathing, clapping and vocalizing of patterns such as "Hee Hee Ha Ha Ha." Then we walked around the room and engaged one another with playful greetings and fake laughter. By the end of the hour, we were all genuinely laughing and we left the class feeling relaxed and uplifted.

This type of program is not everyone's cup of tea, yet for me the takeaway was that I should laugh more—I should lighten up. At times, the seriousness and daily grind of self-care can zap my sense of humor and I am sure you've felt the same way. But, if we think of laughter as another step in our BE CLEAR Method to living with bronchiectasis, it seems less frivolous and more integral to our well-being.

The Mayo Clinic (2019) concurs that laughter has many salutary effects and recommends we find ways to laugh regularly. They say laughter can:

- Stimulate organs
- Activate and relieve our stress response
- Improve our immune system
- Relieve pain
- Improve one's mood

So, let's try to benefit from laughter by looking for ways to let loose a guffaw or two during our day! Whether that means clicking over to an online joke site, watching a comedy hour or reminiscing with family and friends, let's seek out opportunities to laugh.

Having grandchildren and watching them run around and be silly reminds me of how good it is to be present in the moment and enjoy life. My friends with pets have a similar experience watching the fun-loving antics of their cats and dogs. So, whatever our source of laughter, and, yes, even if it makes us cough, let's remember it nourishes the body and spirit. This leads us to the second "E" in *The BE CLEAR Method to Living with Bronchiectasis*—Eating and Drinking. But first let's have a little talk about that annoying problem some of us have while laughing and coughing—urinary incontinence.

Bronchi-X-tra
Stress Urinary Incontinence

Stress urinary incontinence is the unintentional leakage of urine caused by laughing, coughing, blowing your nose, sneezing, jumping, running and lifting heavy objects. The condition can cause social isolation and even depression as some people avoid social situations out of fear of leakage.

Stress incontinence is more prevalent in women, especially older women who have been pregnant, are overweight, have a history of constipation or have a chronic cough. These factors can put pressure on the pelvic floor and cause muscles to weaken. This weakening means the bladder and the bowel and, for women, the uterus, no longer have the support they need.

The good news is that pelvic floor exercises, also known as Kegels, can strengthen the hammock of muscles from the pubic bone to the tailbone. Learning to squeeze and lift these small muscles while relaxing the larger ones is challenging, but practice can help prevent leakage. Pelvic exercises are subtle and you can do them anytime. While waiting for the bus, sitting in the doctor's office or even taking a walk, you can strengthen your pelvic floor!

Thankfully, some therapists specialize in pelvic floor health and can work with you to assess your particular issues and design a treatment plan for you.

Chapter 5

E is for Eating and Drinking

> *Pull up a chair. Take a taste. Come join us. Life is so endlessly delicious.*
>
> RUTH REICHL

> *Food is fuel and not a solution to anything other than giving your body nutrients.*
>
> GABRIELLE REESE (CHAMPION VOLLEYBALL PLAYER)

When I attended my first bronchiectasis patient conference, I couldn't help but notice how thin most attendees were. As we mingled and became acquainted, I heard the repeated concern about a lack of energy. I wondered if maybe they weren't eating enough. But then, during the conference I was surprised to see them pulling baggies of nuts, crackers and chocolates from their bags, some even washing down their goodies with supplemental nutrition drinks. I thought, how could they be so underweight if they were eating such high-calorie foods?!

I later learned that their thinness is caused by several factors including loss of appetite, early satiety, nausea and fatigue. Furthermore, the drugs they take often adversely affect their taste buds, rendering food tasteless or, in some cases, foul-tasting. There is also an increased need for calories when fighting infection as damaged lungs work exceptionally hard to breathe, cough and remove hypersecretions. This exertion causes some to burn through their calories quickly and become underweight. When this occurs, breathing, clearing mucus and performing daily activities become more difficult.

Ideally, we want to be in a healthy weight zone. The U.S. National Institute of Health defines this as having a Body Mass Index (a calculation based on height and weight) between 18.5 and 24.9. If we are undernourished and burning through fat and muscle, our bodies are functioning in emergency mode. In this state, we will not have sufficient energy to support us throughout the day, much less do the vital work of deep breathing, exercise and airway clearance. Registered Dietitian Nutritionist Michelle MacDonald, who specializes in pulmonary disease, prefers a BMI closer to 21 so that the individual may be better able to weather bouts of illness and exacerbations. MacDonald also recommends a high protein diet that includes healthy fats as well as carbohydrates. She believes that eating four to five small meals of all food groups—protein, fats and carbohydrates—is best. And eat that jelly donut if you want it! MacDonald just asks that you enjoy it after nourishing yourself with a healthy meal (personal communication, February 12, 2021).

By now, you might have noticed that I am driving home the point "thin is not in" when it comes to bronchiectasis. If you have spent years yo-yo dieting, then quickly shedding pounds might feel like a welcomed perk of our disease. It's not. Low body weight is associated with a poor BE prognosis. In light of this, I highly recommend you work with a registered dietitian nutritionist to review your eating habits, food preferences and concerns.

In 2020 I took my own advice and had a month's worth of virtual consultations. I eat a mainly vegan diet, so my objective was to double-check that I was getting enough protein, vitamins and minerals. As a health educator, I already had the basics down, but I approached the inquiry with an open mind. The nutritionist and I used an online app and for several weeks I snapped photos of my meals and uploaded them with an ingredients list. I enjoyed the process and we were able to make some improvements to my diet. Most importantly, I felt reassured I was eating well and providing my body with the nourishment it needs to heal.

If your insurance does not cover nutritional consulting, or you prefer to approach the topic on your own, then Harvard School of Public Health's *The Nutrition Source* is an excellent place to learn more about dos and don'ts. Below, I also share some tips and tricks to maintain good nutrition and stay within a healthy weight range. I hope these suggestions are useful and get you thinking about what you can do to ensure you are eating optimally.

EIGHT TIPS TO HEALTHY EATING AND DRINKING

1. Stock Your Shelves, Refrigerator, Freezer and Spice Rack with Good Stuff

Have the ingredients for your go-to meals available in your home. For those who work, are feeling poorly or have other responsibilities, this is not always easy. However, many people do achieve their goal of eating healthy home-cooked meals daily and you can too if you commit to it and plan. The first step is to make a "basics" shopping list that includes all the shelf, refrigerator and freezer ingredients you use regularly. Double up on shelf and freezer items if you have space. If you don't relish cooking every day, purchase ingredients for batch recipes such as soups, stews and casseroles. Be sure to have a lot of storage containers so when you make a pot of soup or stew, you can portion it out, put a couple of containers in the fridge and freeze the rest.

I was never one to freeze food. I prefer to have freshly cooked meals. However, if we want to take control of our eating, having frozen prepared meals is tremendously helpful. For example, if you are a hot food lover like me, a salad for lunch or dinner is not always satisfying. But when I add a bowl of soup to my meal and a piece of dark chocolate for dessert—then I have a feast! As Lidia Bastianich, the famous Italian cookbook author, says, "make your refrigerator or freezer like a treasure chest."

I love soup. Years ago, while living in Italy, an Italian friend taught me how to make the best minestrone and even now, I make it regularly. (See Franca's Minestrone recipe at the end of this chapter.) When I have no desire to cook, I pull a container from the freezer to use in various ways. I may add pasta or rice or pour the thick soup over a baked potato, but mostly I enjoy it just the way it is and with a side salad. This might not be your idea of the most delicious meal in the world, but I'm sure you have a favorite. Go with it. Use it as your meal planning base and change things up by adding other ingredients to it.

If it is difficult for you to shop regularly, consider using your local grocery store's shopping and delivery service. With this type of service, you cannot choose each apple or check expiration dates, and there could be a delivery fee, but when you prepare your own meals, you know what you are eating. However, if your goal is to gain weight and you don't want to cook, then feel free to order in or dine out at your favorite restaurants. In other words, as a nutritional consultant might say, "Just eat!"

2. Cook When You Have the Energy and the Interest

Try to prepare your meals when you have energy and can enjoy the process. Cooking can be creative, and some of us who spend lots of time on self-care might not have many other opportunities to let our creative juices flow. Check out online recipes or buy a cookbook to learn how to make new dishes. Don't forget to leave time for cleanup. Nothing is more of a turn-off to meal preparation than feeling exhausted by the resulting piles of pots and pans to wash and put away. Over time, you will become more efficient in your cooking, make less mess and feel jazzed knowing you are going the extra mile in your commitment to healthy eating.

3. Hit All Your Senses

Both Japanese and Indian cooking are based on the concept that to be appetizing, food should entice the five senses—sight, smell, taste, feel and sound. That's not to say every meal needs to be a Broadway show on a plate, but if you suffer from a poor appetite, you will want to give this some thought. Case in point, a salad with romaine lettuce, cucumbers, and potatoes might contain ingredients you like, but it lacks color and pizzazz. Throw in a handful of red cabbage, some crunchy carrot slices and yellow peppers and then the salad is singing your song.

The importance of eating colorful fruits and vegetables is not just an aesthetic one. The phrase "eating the rainbow" suggests that fruits and vegetables of different colors provide us with a variety of nutrients and health benefits. To have the most nutritious diet, add color to your meal by putting kale in your mac and cheese or assorted roasted veggies on your pizza.

4. Tread Lightly with Trigger Foods

Many of us with BE have sensitive, reactive airways. Certain foods, because of their physical or chemical makeup, can bring about a coughing spell. Coughing while eating can cause liquids and food particles to be aspirated into the lungs. Introducing this foreign matter into the airways leads to more inflammation, tissue damage, infection and mucus. Some of my triggers are astringent food and drink such as lemons and vinegar. Bagels are another problem as their hard crust can irritate the back of my throat and make me cough.

Like with coughing triggers, observe which foods increase mucus and avoid them or eat them sparingly. With that said, be careful about eliminating entire food groups like dairy and gluten unless you are absolutely sure they are causing issues. These foods have essential nutrients and calories and an overly restrictive diet is not advisable.

Some foods might trigger gastric reflux. Common culprits are fatty foods, tomato sauce, carbonated and caffeinated drinks, alcohol and sadly, chocolate. Although it is hard to believe, GERD can be silent, meaning that there are no symptoms. Yet, even without symptoms, acid and non-acid stomach contents can make their way up the esophagus and into the lungs. It is a good idea to be tested for GERD, but regardless, simple lifestyle modifications such as not eating within three hours of your bedtime and elevating the head of the bed might be beneficial.

5. Walk to Pop Your "Digestion Clutch"

I am a sucker for period films like Jane Austen's *Pride and Prejudice*, featuring women walking miles to visit neighboring estates. Nowadays, to motivate ourselves to walk, we resort to using step-counting apps on our phones. If you have digestive issues, and many with BE do, I encourage you to do whatever it takes to motivate yourself to go for an after-dinner constitutional. It can help kick your digestion into gear and reduce coughing and shortness of breath.

6. Stay hydrated but not over-hydrated

Dr. Gwen Huitt, at National Jewish Health, believes that consuming too much liquid can cause reflux and recommends no more than six ounces per hour throughout the day. This includes foods like soups, smoothies and yogurt. (Dell, 2018).

If you are looking to gain weight, caloric drinks like milkshakes and supplemental nutrition drinks are best. Also, limit mealtime non-calorie drinks as they can fill you up before you've had enough to eat. Of course, you should have some water available if you need to wash something down or if you start coughing.

7. Keep a Food Diary, maybe

As I mentioned, I wrote down what I ate in a food diary for a while. Keeping a record of my daily meals and snacks helped the nutritionist look for deficiencies in my diet. Furthermore, it made me more aware of my eating habits and whether any foods or situations caused congestion or coughing. If you are not working with a nutritionist and already feel like you are doing a million self-care practices and the thought of a food diary is like nails on a chalkboard, then don't do it. Just think about what you eat and how it makes you feel and see if you can come up with improvements.

8. Be Mindful While Eating

Being mindful means not thinking about what happened in the past or what could occur in the future. Enjoying the food on our plate, bite by bite is one way to be in the moment. Savoring the colors, textures, tastes and aroma of our food will make it more satisfying. Unfortunately, we frequently deprive ourselves of this focused, meditative experience by eating while watching television or using computers and phones. We may blame our food if we cough or experience indigestion but our overloaded minds could actually be causing the discomfort. How do we learn to be in the moment when nowadays we are so used to multi-tasking that it feels strange to just sit and eat? The next two chapters address unlocking our innate ability to be present and to heal.

Bronchi-X-tra
Franca's Minestrone

1 large onion, chopped
5 cloves of garlic, minced
1/3 cup of extra virgin olive oil
½ medium cabbage, thinly sliced
2 medium zucchini diced
2 medium carrots diced
1 cup of mushrooms, sliced
1 cup of fresh spinach, chopped
1 28 oz can of crushed San Marzano tomatoes
1 19 oz can of cannellini beans (or freshly cooked beans)
32 ounces of vegetable broth
32 ounces of water (or vegetable broth for more flavor)
3 basil leaves, chopped
Salt and pepper to taste

Optional
3 medium potatoes, diced
1/3 stick of butter
2 tablespoons of Worcestershire sauce (for more flavor)
8 oz of pasta such as orzo
1 cup of freshly grated parmesan cheese (nutritional yeast is a good vegan substitute)

Fry the onions and garlic in olive oil in a large pot, stirring constantly. When they are translucent, add the cabbage. Cook on medium until soft. Add all other ingredients except for the pasta and cheese. If needed, fill the pot with more water to cover the vegetables. Simmer for one hour or longer if you want a thicker soup with a richer flavor. Cook pasta separately. Add pasta and cheese to individual bowls. Finish with a sprinkling of fresh chopped basil and a drizzle of olive oil. For a thicker soup, cool and then blend half of the pot in a blender and add it back in with the other half. Makes 8 servings.

Chapter 6

A is for Alternative Therapies

Far from being simply the absence of disease, health is a dynamic and harmonious equilibrium of all the elements and forces making up and surrounding a human being.

ANDREW WEIL

A lternative therapies refer to wellness services that are not part of traditional western medicine. Also known as complementary medicine, this care includes Ayurveda, Traditional Chinese Medicine (TCM), chiropractic, homeopathy, yoga, massage, meditation and various forms of what is broadly called energy work. These services are frequently available in hospitals, community centers and privately-owned businesses like yoga studios.

Some modalities, such as acupuncture and chiropractic care, you experience as a passive participant. Other therapies like Reiki, Jin Shin Jyutsu and massage are administered by a practitioner who can also teach you a simplified version to perform on yourself. Then there are practices like Tai Chi, yoga and meditation that you can do independently. You might have a Tai Chi or yoga teacher guide you, but you are the one who moves through the different positions.

Learning about alternative therapies can be fascinating and over the past forty years I have sampled many of them. Here I'll share several of these experiences including acupuncture, Jin Shin Jyutsu and yoga. If you prefer to stick to a more traditional wellness approach—healthy eating and exercise, I support you. If you should want to dabble in healing methods, first get your doctor's approval. Then ask friends and family for input and see what is available in your community. You can also search national certification sites to find practitioners in your area.

The research that backs up the benefits of alternative therapy for people with chronic disease and, more specifically, lung disease, is inconclusive and not easily verifiable. For example, if a study shows benefits from one type of yoga, it does not mean another kind of yoga will have the same effect. Even without unequivocal results, 38 percent of adults are using some form of alternative medicine (American Thoracic Society [ATS], 2017). National Jewish Health acknowledges that these non-traditional practices can benefit some people with lung disease. They say, "along with an appropriate medical treatment plan, additional therapies may provide relief to those suffering from chronic lung disease. You should recognize that there is not one method of treatment that is right for everyone and work closely with your physician to figure out what works best for you." (National Jewish Health, n.d.)

I cannot say alternative practices have helped my lungs heal or boosted my immunity. However, I can say that when I receive a treatment or practice therapies on my own, I usually feel a profound sense of calm. As with the deep breathing exercises discussed in *BE CLEAR's* first chapter, these therapies quiet the sympathetic nervous system by relaxing the body and soothing the mind. Worry and fear decrease in the moment, sometimes with long-lasting effects.

Doctors have never asked whether I use alternative health practices. Instead, they ask me how I feel and about symptoms. Then, we review test results and treatment options. All of this updating leaves little time for inquiring about non-traditional adjunctive care. Moreover, with scant evidence-based research and the broad range of alternative therapies available, many doctors are not comfortable endorsing alternative modalities.

All the same, you might wish to share your alternative care practices with your medical team. Even if your doctors stop short of vouching for your practices, they could have suggestions. For example, if you have GERD and do yoga, your doctor may recommend you not eat before class, as in many positions your head is lower than your stomach which could cause reflux. Or, if your medications are affecting your balance, your doctor could suggest tai chi or yoga classes to improve your stability and prevent falling. As for myself, I enjoy sharing with doctors what I am doing to promote healing. It feels like more of a partnership this way and gives them a broader, more holistic sense of who I am. It says, "I trust you as my doctor but I am a well-informed, take-charge sort of person and I want you to know that about me."

ACUPUNCTURE

Anything that has been around for a long time earns my respect. Whether we are talking about 20,000-year-old cave drawings or ancient health practices like acupuncture, they have withstood the test of time. Acupuncture is described by the National Institute of Health (NIH) as a Chinese health system that has been around for more than 2,500 years. Its tenets are complex and difficult to summarize, but in a nutshell, Traditional Chinese Medicine (TCM), of which acupuncture is one component, views the human body and its relationship to the world as one of harmony involving oppositional forces, yin and yang. When the flow of energy known as qi (pronounced *chee*) is disrupted, "dis-ease" and unwellness can result. Acupuncture stimulates points along body pathways called meridians to encourage the full functioning of our endocrine, digestive, cardiovascular and immune systems.

NYU Langone Health, where I go for my medical care, offers integrative health services including acupuncture. Their website states that acupuncture may help ease stress, anxiety, and acute and chronic pain (NYU Langone Health, n.d.). I first tried acupuncture in 1998 when I moved to New York City and was going through a difficult period in my life. I was stressed and at times incapacitated by severe low-back pain and headaches. I went to Chinatown and saw an acupuncturist who inserted thin needles into my body, barely penetrating my skin. I had a half dozen treatments and found that I experienced relief from my pain which allowed me to ease off ibuprofen and resume my regular stretching program.

I have continued to get acupuncture from time to time for ailments including an injured shoulder, digestive issues and bronchiectasis. Recently I went to an acupuncture school clinic for treatment. As soon as the student and teacher placed micro-fine needles along my arms and across my chest, I felt mucus gurgle up. Several times during the treatment I needed to clear my throat of what was being released from my lungs. Throughout the day I had a feeling of well-being and was not at all congested, even though I had not cleared my airways before acupuncture. In the evening, when I nebulized saline and used my Aerobika, there was nothing to clear. For me, acupuncture continues to be a useful therapy.

JIN SHIN JYUTSU®

Jin Shin Jyutsu (Jin Shin) is an ancient Japanese healing practice passed down from generation to generation until it was lost to obscurity. In the early 1900s, Juro Murai, a Japanese man with a life-threatening illness, in his quest to heal himself rediscovered Jin Shin in the sacred Kojiki texts, the oldest books of Japanese history and culture. This practice was then brought to the United States in the 1950s. Jin Shin is based on a theory of stagnation in the energy pathways, similar to acupuncture. Instead of using needles as in acupuncture, the practitioner's hands (or our own hands when we do Jin Shin self-care) are used to move energy and free up blockages. While not as well-known as energy work like Reiki and reflexology, Jin Shin practitioners are in many U.S. states and worldwide.

According to a discussion between Alexis Brink, founder of the Jin Shin Institute in New York City and Deepak Chopra, the well-known guru of alternative healing therapies, he felt lighter after his sessions with Alexis. He also felt his body return to its natural homeostasis (defined as a balance in the body regardless of external factors) and self-regulation which is when natural healing occurs (The Chopra Well, 2019).

I love Jin Shin because I can be treated by a practitioner or do it on myself. When I first discovered Jin Shin two years ago, I saw Alexis weekly to test the work's benefits. Being the skeptic and mad scientist I am, I would experiment by sometimes doing airway clearance before my session and sometimes not. Regardless, within ten minutes of getting on Alexis' table (always face up and with clothes on) and having her place her hands on my body, I would start to unblock. Just like with acupuncture, I would feel lung gurgles and the need to cough. By the end of the session, my body would tingle and a sense of well-being would wash over me.

As much as I enjoy sessions with Alexis, for me, it is all about self-care. I do not want to be dependent on anyone to "fix me." After attending several self-care workshops and with Alexis' book, *The Art of Jin Shin* nearby for reference, I feel confident in my self-care practice. Whether it is to fall back to sleep when I wake too early or for better airway clearance, I use my hands to move my body's energy and access the help I need at that moment.

YOGA

Yogic philosophies and practices can be traced back thousands of years, similar to acupuncture and Jin Shin's ancient origins. The word "yoga" comes from the ancient Indian Sanskrit language and means to yoke or bring together. By joining and balancing opposing energies in our body as well as the mind and spirit, yoga fosters better health through harmony. Many think yoga is strictly a physical program involving warrior poses, balance challenges and twists. While these asanas (poses) stretch and strengthen our bodies, they are just one aspect of a full yoga practice. If you go through a physical routine without attention to your breath or mind, you miss out on the deeper benefits of a more holistic yogic experience.

Completing a yoga certification program fifteen years ago was life-changing. I spent a month with aspiring yoga teachers, many much younger than me who excelled at gravity-defying feats that were too taxing for my middle-aged body. I learned to be happy by just being present and doing my best. This self-acceptance has helped me in every aspect of my life, especially with my current challenge of managing bronchiectasis.

If you find a good yoga teacher locally or online, I hope you will enjoy the practice as much as I do. Do not get down on yourself if you cannot be a human pretzel like the person next to you or in the video. If you encounter challenges in the process, such as acid reflux, tender wrists or arthritic hips, you can ask your teacher for modifications. When doing an online class, if a pose does not feel comfortable, sit and focus on your breath until you are able to do the next pose. Or, if that form of yoga does not seem right for you, choose a different form. There are many types of yoga and many teaching styles. I am confident that with a little experimentation, you will find a good match.

Meditation, often included in a yoga practice, is another versatile and effective alternative therapy in and of itself. As Sharon Salzberg, co-founder of the Insight Meditation Society says, "meditation is the ultimate mobile device; you can use it anywhere, anytime, unobtrusively." (Salzberg, 2011, p.21) In the following chapter, I'll share ways to develop a meditation practice to quiet the mind, relax the body and allow natural healing to occur.

Bronchi-X-tra
How to Begin a Self-Care Alternative Therapy Exploration

Although each alternative therapy has its own underlying philosophy, they often have much in common. Most notably, all use the breath as an integral part of the practice. For practices where the participant is in motion, like Tai Chi, Yoga, Qigong, and walking meditation, the breathwork and movement are often coordinated. Practices that do not involve motion, such as Reiki, Jin Shin Jyutsu and seated meditation, also use the breath to promote the natural flow of life force throughout the body and to calm the mind.

Not sure which one to try or how to decide? I suggest starting slowly and not overcommitting. Choose an introductory class to learn the basics and be able to practice on your own. Also, considerate the following options:

- **Private Instruction** (in-person or online)

    ◊ Provides personalized instruction addressing an individual's health status and preferences
    ◊ Flexible scheduling
    ◊ Can be expensive

- **Group Classes** (in-person or live streaming)

    ◊ Can be an opportunity to socialize (perhaps attend with a friend)
    ◊ Best if conveniently located near your home or workplace
    ◊ Can be expensive
    ◊ Often cannot address an individual's health status and preferences
    ◊ Coughing during class may be a concern
    ◊ Less expensive than one-on-one instruction

- **Apps with recorded sessions**

    ◊ Lots of choices
    ◊ Flexibility to participate on your own schedule
    ◊ Do not address an individual's health status and preferences
    ◊ Inexpensive

Experiment—Be Open—Have Fun!!

Chapter 7

R is for Relaxation, Rest and Sleep

> *Almost everything will work again if you unplug it for a few minutes, including you.*
>
> ANNE LAMOTT

> *There is a time for many words, and there is also a time for sleep.*
>
> HOMER

R for Relaxation, Rest and Sleep comes at the end of the Method, but it does not mean it is less important than everything else we have discussed. Quite the contrary, it seals in the juices from our self-care labors and is vital to healing. Relaxation, which is freeing the mind and body from tension, can be achieved by walking in nature, participating in an enjoyable pastime or through breathing practices and meditation.

RELAXATION AND MEDITATION

Andy Puddicombe, author of *The Headspace Guide to Meditation and Mindfulness*, likens meditation to riding a bike. When we first learn to bike ride, it might be just for fun. Later, we might ride for exercise or as a means of transportation. Meditation works with the same versatility. It might initially improve one's focus in school. Later, it can reduce the stress of juggling work and family responsibilities. Personally, I find that meditation teaches me to stay committed to self-care and not become demoralized by fearful thinking.

Meditating by repeating a sound or word

Dr. Herbert Benson, founder of Harvard's Mind/Body Institute, published a ground-breaking book in 1975 called *The Relaxation*

Response. Based on a study of meditators with high blood pressure, the book stated that their blood pressure dropped significantly in the weeks they meditated regularly. As soon as they stopped, their blood pressure went back up. Benson demystified meditation, describing it as an innate survival mechanism we all possess to counteract the fight-or-flight response when in overdrive. According to Benson, a process he named the Relaxation Response occurs while meditating and is a "built-in, inducible, physiological state of quietude (that has) the ability to heal and rejuvenate our bodies." (Benson, 1975, p.157)

Benson found that the two essential steps to eliciting the Relaxation Response are:

- Repeating a sound, word, prayer or doing a repetitive physical activity (such as walking, swimming or yoga)
- Disregarding thoughts that inevitably come to your mind and returning to your repetition.

When I was initiated into Transcendental Meditation (TM) in 1974, I was given a two-syllable mantra (a special word with vibrational qualities) to say repeatedly during my twenty-minute meditation. While inhaling I would say the first syllable and while exhaling, the second. If you do not go through a formal meditation program like TM, you can use "so-hum" as a mantra. So-hum meditation has existed in India for ages. The Sanskrit words "so" means "I am" and "hum" means "that." It is an affirmation of being a part of a larger whole, described as universal consciousness.

Find a quiet place to sit (when you get more comfortable with meditating, ambient noise will be less distracting) and say "so" with your inhalation and "hum" with your exhalation. As thoughts float into your mind, and they will, just say to yourself, "I'm thinking" and gently push the thoughts aside. Repeat the process whenever necessary, always returning to your so-hum mantra afterward. Start with five minutes and, if you wish, lengthen your meditation when you are ready. In time, you may enjoy meditating in the morning and then a second time later in the day.

Walking Meditation

If sitting for meditation does not appeal to you or you want to mix it up, try meditating while walking. The Vietnamese Zen Monk, Thich Nhat Hanh, advocates adding this movement-based practice to your self-care. It is a way to connect with the earth and tap into the power of nature.

REST

It is important for some people with chronic conditions to put their feet up to rest during the day. Many with bronchiectasis are extremely tired. This exhaustion can be caused by many things including shortness of breath, our body fighting the disease, exercise, airway clearance and poor sleep quality, but regardless, it is a serious issue that cannot be ignored.

As difficult as it is for some to stop several times during the day to "take a time out," it is essential for optimal health. Sitting or lying down when you feel your energy waning is an important way to manage your self-care. If you can nap, all the better. Napping, sometimes thought of as a guilty pleasure, can be a necessity for those with a chronic disease. Dr. Ilene Rosen, a researcher from the University of Pennsylvania's School of Medicine, says that while there is no consensus on the ideal duration of a nap, she believes that a ten to twenty-minute nap is ideal to recharge (Reddy, 2013). Just as with the other steps in the BE CLEAR Method, the best way to know what is optimal for you is to experiment.

The downside to taking daytime naps is that napping might make you less sleepy at nighttime. I find if I read in the afternoon, often my eyes get tired and I'll doze for ten to fifteen minutes. The resulting power nap is refreshing and gives me a second wind for the late afternoon, sometimes with the benefit of being able to add in a half-hour of early evening exercise. On the rare occasion I sleep for over thirty minutes, I wake up feeling groggy and can have trouble falling asleep at my regular bedtime.

SLEEP

The American Sleep Apnea Association (n.d.) states that sleep is "… indeed as vital as the air we breathe and the food we eat, especially for those with chronic diseases or compromised immune systems." Taking into consideration the seriousness of adequate sleep (often defined as seven hours or more for adults 18-60 years of age) it is alarming that fifty to seventy million adults in the U.S. report sleep-related problems (American Sleep Apnea Association, n.d.). Should we view our sleep deprivation as a cultural issue? Are we hard-coded with a desire to be productive and have too much on our plates? Are our electronic devices fueling the need to "take care of one more thing"? I think so. Societal attitudes and electronic connectivity can foster the idea that we aren't "in the game" unless we are always on the go.

The importance of sleep is undeniable. After all, would our miraculously intricate bodies waste so much time sleeping if it were not so important? Scientists confirm that a lot is happening while we are in deep slumber. The brain performs checks on all systems and makes sure it is cleaned out of waste matter and in tip-top condition. If we continually skimp on sleep, the brain does not function properly and, especially for people with chronic diseases, this can create a serious situation. "We all want to push the system, to get the most out of our lives, and sleep gets in the way," says pulmonologist and sleep researcher Dr. Sigrid Veasey. "But we need to know how far we can really push that system and get away with it." (Park, 2014)

Twenty years ago, while studying yoga and Indian yogic health practices called Ayurveda, I was introduced to the concept of ideal sleeping time. Ayurveda health practices state the best time for sleep is from 10 pm to 6 am. This sleep protocol's rationale is that the most desirable, restorative sleep is likely to occur before midnight. With this in mind, I slowly changed my bedtime and inched my way back to a 10 pm lights-out goal.

A 10 pm self-imposed curfew is not for everyone. I have a friend who is a retired actress and, even though she is no longer on Broadway, her body still prefers a late-to-bed, late-to-rise schedule. This night-owl timetable coincides with her individual biological clock, what is known as circadian rhythm. For people, like my friend, who do not go to bed early, the best compromise is to choose the same eight hours for sleeping and maintain that schedule. It's all about creating a habit that your mind and body will respond to. This is the first step of what is often referred to as sleep hygiene. When we talk about sleep hygiene, I am not talking about the crispness of your bed linens. (Although some say it does make a difference in their sleep.) I am referring to the routine you build to usher in a satisfying period of restorative sleep. It is a series of wind-down actions that begin about an hour before your bedtime.

Some possible steps are:

- Turn off your electronic devices or silence them. If possible, remove them from your bedroom.
- Clear your bedroom of unnecessary stuff including piles of laundry, stacks of bills and airway clearance devices.
- If your bed is unmade from day-napping, straighten it out and fluff the pillows.
- Crack the window open to freshen and cool off the room or turn down the heat.
- Dim your bedroom lights.
- Put on some relaxing music.
- Do some light stretching or gentle yoga.
- Massage and moisturize yourself.
- Read a book. Preferably not an e-book but a paper one. Even better if it is a little boring.
- Do some relaxation self-care such as energy work, meditation or foot reflexology.
- Breathe deeply and calmly.

If you get in bed and start coughing and have trouble falling asleep or staying asleep, discuss this issue with your medical team. They might recommend elevating the head of your bed or sleeping on a pillow wedge. Clearing your airways in the evening might also decrease coughing. In some cases, your physician will want you to be tested for sleep apnea, a sleep disorder that can become serious if not addressed. Having to get up to use the bathroom repeatedly during the night can also get in the way of a good night's sleep. Bring this up to your medical team, too. Changes in when you eat and drink and take your medication might mean fewer trips to the bathroom and a better night's sleep.

Remember to practice self-compassion if you do not sleep well. Rather than get down on yourself or become anxious thinking about how you won't sleep well again, use your meditation skills and let those negative thoughts float on by. Remind yourself that your bedtime ritual, while not one hundred percent effective, works.

FINAL THOUGHTS

There is an ancient Japanese art called Kintsugi, which translates to "gold joinery." In this art, broken ceramics are repaired with gold, creating refurbished wares as strong as the old ones. Often showcased as art, their golden scars add both beauty and uniqueness to these vessels.

This is true for us as well. We can mourn the people we once were and feel broken, or we can embrace the beauty of our new reality. Through acceptance, determination and resilience we can continue to be ourselves and inspire others. As my favorite poet and musician Leonard Cohen says in his song, "Anthem":

> *Ring the bells that still can ring,*
> *Forget your perfect offering,*
> *There is a crack in everything,*
> *That's how the light gets in.*

I sincerely hope that *The BE CLEAR Method to Living with Bronchiectasis* is helpful to you. That you "ring the bells" and remain proud and fearless, safe in the knowledge that you have the tools, support and confidence to face the challenges of bronchiectasis. That you let your unique spirit shine out while allowing the care from those around you, including the bronchiectasis community, shine in. Let us continue to learn and experiment together. We have a condition that has not been well-understood and is now gaining attention in the medical community. These are exciting times for us.

REFERENCES

Addrizzo-Harris, D., Barrios, C., Candotra, S., Sagar, M., & Sheda, G., Jr. (2017). *Living Well with Bronchiectasis* [Brochure]. The Chest Foundation. foundation.chestnet.org/wp-content/uploads/2020/05/Bronchiectasis-Living-Well.pdf

American Sleep Apnea Association. (n.d.). *Sleep-Wake Disorders.* Retrieved April 14, 2021, from sleepapnea.org/sleep-health/the-state-of-sleephealth-in-america

American Thoracic Society. (2017). Integrative Medicine (Complementary and Alternative Medicine) for the Lungs. *American Journal of Respiratory and Critical Care Medicine, 195*(11), 21-22. https://doi.org/10.1164/rccm.19511P21

Benson, H. (1975). *The Relaxation Response.* Avon.

Berk, L. S., Tan, S. A., Fry, W. F., Napier, B. J., Lee, J. W., Hubbard, R. W., Lewis, J. E., and Ebay, W. C. (1989, December). Neuroendocrine and stress hormone changes during mirthful laughter. *American Journal of*

*Medical Sciences, 298(*6), 390-396. https://doi.org/10.1097/00000441-198912000-00006

Chalmers, J. D., Aliberti, S., & Blasi, F. (2015). Management of bronchiectasis in adults. *European Respiratory Journal, 45*(5), 1446-1462. https://doi.org/10.1183/09031936.00119114

Chalmers, J. D., Sibila, O. (2020). Happy Birthday, Bronchiectasis: 200 Years of Targeting Mucus. *American Journal of Respiratory and Critical Care Medicine, 201*(6), 639-640. https://doi.org/10.1164/rccm.201911-2261ED

Colburn, D. (1986, October 21). Norman Cousins, Still Laughing. *The Washington Post.* washingtonpost.com/archive/lifestyle/wellness/1986/10/21/norman-cousins-still-laughing/e17f23cb-3e8c-4f58-b907-2dcd00326e22

Dell, B. (2018, March 15). *7 tips for Preventing Reflux and Aspiration.* Cystic Fibrosis News Today. cysticfibrosisnewstoday.com/2018/03/15/7-tips-preventing-reflux-aspiration

Department of Health and Human Services. (2019). *Executive Summary: Physical Activity Guidelines for Americans* (2nd ed.). health.gov/sites/default/files/2019-10/PAG_ExecutiveSummary.pdf

Federation of American Societies for Experimental Biology. (2010, April 26). Body's response to repetitive laughter is similar to the effect of repetitive exercise, study finds. *ScienceDaily.* https://www.sciencedaily.com/releases/2010/04/100426113058.htm

Greenspan, N. (2017). *Ultimate Pulmonary Wellness.* BookBaby.

Hill, A. T., Sullivan, A.L., Chalmers, J. D., De Soyza, A., Elborn, J. S., Floto, R. A., Grillo, L., Gruffydd-Jones, K., Harvey, A., Haworth, C. S., Hiscocks, E., Hurst, J. R., Johnson, C., Kelleher, W. P., Bedi, P., Payne,

K., Saleh, H., Screaton, N. J., Loebinger, M. R. (2019). British Thoracic Society Guideline for bronchiectasis in adults. *Thorax, 74*(1), 1-69. http://dx.doi.org/10.1136/thoraxjnl-2018-212463

Mayo Clinic (2019, April 5). Str*ess relief from laughter? It's no joke.* mayoclinic.org/healthy-lifestyle/stress-management/in-depth/stress-relief/art-20044456

Monahganmed. (n.d.). *Aerobika OPEP.* Retrieved April 14, 2021, from https://www.monaghanmed.com/Aerobika/

National Jewish Health. (n.d.). *Alternative Therapies.* Retrieved April 14, 2021, from nationaljewish.org/conditions/medications/asthma-medications/alternative

NTM Info & Research [NTMir]. (2020, November 6). *Airway Clearance* [Video]. Youtube. youtube.com/watch?v=L-EHohMe7II

NYU Langone Health. (n.d.). *Outpatient Integrative Health Services.* Retrieved April 14, 2021, from nyulangone.org/patient-family-support/integrative-health-services-for-adults/outpatient-integrative-health-services

Park, A. (2014, September 11). The Power of Sleep. *Time.* https://time.com/3326565/the-power-of-sleep

Peterson, L. A. (2017, March 23) *Decrease stress by using breath.* Mayo Clinic. mayoclinic.org/healthy-lifestyle/stress-management/in-depth/decrease-stress-by-using-your-breath/art-20267197

Qi, Q., Li, T., Li, J. C., & Li, Y. (2015). Association of body mass index with disease severity and prognosis in patients with non-cystic fibrosis bronchiectasis. *Brazilian Journal of Medical and Biological Research, 48*(8), 715–724. https://doi.org/10.1590/1414-431X20154135

Reddy, S. (2013, September 2). The Perfect Nap: Sleeping is a Mix of Art and Science. *The Wall Street Journal*. wsj.com/articles/the-perfect-nap-sleeping-is-a-mix-of-art-and-science-1378155665

Salzberg, S. (2011). *Real Happiness: The Power of Meditation*. Workman Publishing Company.

The Chopra Well. (2019, June 22). *The Art of Jin Shin: A conversation with Alexis Brink*. [Video]. YouTube. youtube.com/watch?v=h2-IAMsvdik

Weycker, D., Hansen, G. L., & Seifert, F. D. (2017). Prevalence and incidence of noncystic fibrosis bronchiectasis among US adults in 2013. *Chronic Respiratory Disease*, *14*(4), 377–384. https://doi.org/10.1177/1479972317709649

RESOURCES

BE CLEAR with Bronchiectasis *
https://letsbecleartoday.com

Bronchiectasis Info and Research
https://bronchiectasisinfo.org

Bronchiectasis Toolbox (Australia)
https://bronchiectasis.com.au

The CHEST Foundation
https://foundation.chestnet.org/lung-health-a-z/bronchiectasis

The Bronchiectasis and NTM Initiative
https://bronchiectasisandntminitiative.org

Patient Priorities (European Lung Foundation and the European
Respiratory Society)
https://europeanlunginfo.org/bronchiectasis

British Lung Foundation
https://blf.org.uk/support-for-you/bronchiectasis

*For up-to-date bronchiectasis information, research, blog posts and more about my personal story, please visit the *BE CLEAR with Bronchiectasis, LLC* website: https://www.LetsBeClearToday.com

BE CLEAR DAILY EXERCISE CHECKLIST*

Day	Activity	Time of day	Duration	Airway clearance before or after	Feeling before exercise	Feeling after exercise	Mucus production notes	Notes
Monday								
Tuesday								
Wednesday								
Thursday								
Friday								
Saturday								
Sunday								

*The purpose of this checklist is to use the recorded information to better understand how exercise impacts your feeling of well-being. Also, to gain insight into the relationship between exercise and airway clearance.

ACKNOWLEDGMENTS

I would like to acknowledge the clinicians and researchers who have chosen bronchiectasis and Nontuberculous Mycobacterial Lung Disease as their professional focus. Your dedication and willingness to guide us through uncertain waters have inspired me to contribute in my small way. I would particularly like to thank Dr. Doreen Addrizzo-Harris and the other excellent clinicians and researchers who care for me at NYU Langone in New York City. I am fortunate beyond belief.

A big thank you to Dr. Colin Swenson and Dr. Wendi Drummond for *NTMTalk*, their excellent educational podcast series on bronchiectasis and NTM infections. The time and energy you selflessly put into your series motivated me to give this book my all.

I would also like to thank Dr. James D. Chalmers from the University of Dundee, Scotland for his research and enthusiasm for sharing valuable information on bronchiectasis in conferences and seminars. I have learned so much from you.

There are too many other researchers to list here; however, I have to give a shout-out to Dr. Joseph O. Falkinham, III. I know that I have emailed you more times than I would like to admit, and others in the BE and

NTM communities have too. You always answer our questions, even the follow-ups to the follow-ups.

Thank you to Michelle MacDonald, RDN and Cheryl Torres, RRT for reviewing chapters on their areas of expertise and giving me constructive input. I am grateful for your willingness to take time from your busy lives to help me. I take full responsibility for those chapters and I hope you are happy with what I wrote.

I also want to thank Insmed, Trudell Medical International and other companies within the lung disease arena for their research. Those of us with BE can breathe a little easier knowing you are working to improve our lives. Also, a heartfelt thank you to the nonprofit NTM Info & Research and its companion website Bronchiectasis Info and Research, for keeping us up-to-date on issues that impact our health.

To Debbie, my mentor and friend who explained bronchiectasis to me when I was first diagnosed and, when I became emotional, assured me that I would be okay. Because of you, I saw my path forward more clearly.

To Carmela, I thank you many times over for reading my guide as I wrote it and, in your gentle way, making me a better writer.

Thank you to Judy and Bernie for your encouragement and friendship.

To my long-time friend, Nancy, thank you for reassuring me that BE CLEAR is authentic to my voice and spirit.

To my bronchi-sisters, Kristina, Marcia, Pooja, Fernanda, Maria, Jan, Terry, Peggy and Kathy, thank you for taking time from your self-care to review my book and share your thoughts.

Thank you to my dear friend of 18 years, Pam Ross, who died from COVID-19. The way you handled your autoimmune disease with such grace and acceptance is a guiding light for me. I won't parachute out of a plane the way you did, but I will try to find joy in everything I do.

To my new friend, Andrée, thank you for allowing me to drop off my manuscript, chapter by chapter, in your mailbox for the fresh ideas that helped me bring the book to a close.

To my over-the-moon supportive sister, Sandy, who is the most enthusiastic person I know. Thank you for always making time to hear my concerns and for brainstorming solutions.

Thank you to my fierce, can-do daughters, Lisa and Daniela. The passion you show for your careers drives me to pursue work that makes me, just like you, hop out of bed in the morning. Thank you for your steadfast support and for my grandchildren, Luna, Solomon, Dario and Dante. Having you guys in my life is why I go the extra lap. I hope to stay healthy and be with you for years to come.

Most of all, I thank my husband, Tony. For over two years, you have listened to me talk about this book, and you read and re-read every word I wrote. Having your intelligent ear and editing skills at my request has been a superpower. It gave me consistent confidence to move forward with this project. I share this accomplishment with you.

ABOUT THE AUTHOR

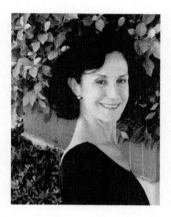

Linda Cooper Esposito lives in New York City with her husband. She enjoys visiting museums, taking long walks around the city, preparing her specialty soups and reading. Her favorite activity is going to Connecticut to see her daughters and grandchildren.

Website: https://www.letsbecleartoday.com

facebook.com/becleartoday

twitter.com/becleartoday

instagram.com/beclearwithbronchiectasis

Printed in Great Britain
by Amazon

74058397R00078